SOTHIS PRESS

Sothis Press aims to completely reimagine the public domain book with an emphasis on universal access to captivatingly designed print editions. We believe that technology will enable every single book ever published to be perpetually accessible in beautiful print form. Sothis is beauty in ubiquity.

www.sothis.press

1 Waterhouse Square, London, ECIN 2ST

The Mighty Curative Powers of Mesmerism

Proved in Upwards of One Hundred and Fifty Cases of Various Diseases

Thomas Capern

SOTHIS PRESS

ISBN 978-1-0368-0212-7

The Mighty Curative Powers of Mesmerism
is in the public domain.

This edition is published by
Sothis Press © 2023. The company
is registered in England and Wales.
The Company Number is 14900389.

THE MIGHTY CURATIVE POWERS OF MESMERISM,

PROVED IN UPWARDS OF

ONE HUNDRED AND FIFTY CASES

OF

Various Diseases.

BY THOMAS CAPERN,

SECRETARY AND RESIDENT SUPERINTENDENT OF THE MESMERIC INFIRMARY.

"Prove all things: hold fast that which is good."
1 *Thes.* v., 21.

London:

H. BAILLIERE, 219, REGENT STREET.

1851.

This little Work

IS DEDICATED TO ALL THOSE

WHO ARE WILLING TO CAST ASIDE THE PRIDE OF

ERUDITION AND TALENT

AND BECOME AS LITTLE CHILDREN,

TO LEARN ALL TRUTH,

AND TO LABOUR FOR THE GOOD OF THEIR

FELLOW-CREATURES.

CONTENTS.

INDEX.

PREFACE.

THE fact of mesmerism having received the most earnest attention from gentlemen of high ability and profound knowledge, and holding the most important situations in society, gives an additional impetus to my desire —humble author as I am—to lay before the world statements of the most undeniable character, derived from my five years experience of the wondrous power of the mesmeric treatment of various diseases. Nearly five years ago I attended a lecture given by the able and excellent Mr. Davey, who had to his great credit risen from the position of a working man to be a lecturer on this important subject; and for his exertions in this holy cause he merits the thanks of his countrymen. At the first lecture I observed great phenomena produced, and, having been favored with a private interview with Mr. Davey, was induced, at the third lecture to ascend the platform; and I assisted at the business by demesmerising one of the persons who had been put into a state of coma. This was sufficient to bring upon myself the most unjust and uncharitable remarks. On further investigating the subject, and after having been favoured with some suggestions from Mr. Davey with respect to the application of mesmerism as a curative agent, I commenced my operations, and was pleased to find some cases in which relief from pain was the result. The first case of importance was that of John Rowden, whom I met accidentally as he was going with difficulty to his labour: and the case is detailed at p. 18—20. Having thus succeeded, I devoted nearly the whole of my time to similar operations on persons of all ages, on the very old and on helpless infants. For thus applying my time and being instrumental in affording relief to my suffering fellow creatures, I was subjected to abuse and insult, even while returning from the sick chambers of those whom disease had brought to the brink of the grave. The titles of *maniac* and *humbug* were bestowed upon me. The term *maniac* I disregarded; but the term *humbug* I did stoutly fling back. However, I was determined to persevere, knowing that the science was based on eternal truth and would prevail and be acknowledged when its calumniators should be utterly forgotten.

Finding it difficult to satisfy the public mind and to

promulgate that such a power existed, I invited the whole of the church clergy, the dissenting ministers, the authorities of the town, the gentry of the parish and neighbourhood, and specially the medical profession, to attend and investigate the phenomena on the 5th of October, 1848. The facts were presented by the introduction of upwards of thirty persons who had received benefit and been cured by my mesmeric manipulations. The individuals, as they presented themselves to the meeting, related in their own language the nature and duration of the disease and the amount of benefit effected by the mesmeric power. The diseases were various; and many of the cases had been discharged from the Exeter Hospital as incurable. At the conclusion of the investigation, which lasted nearly three hours, the Rev. John Spurway moved, and the Rev. Mr. Madgin seconded, a vote of thanks to myself—the reverend gentlemen speaking in the highest terms of the candour and honour of the proceeding, by which every individual case had been boldly subjected to a trying ordeal in the presence of so large a number of well-informed and professional gentlemen. The entire company, a considerable portion of which consisted of ladies connected with the principal families in the neighbourhood, expressed themselves satisfied with the result of the meeting. Amongst those who attended were John Snell, Esq., the mayor, who presided; John Heathcoat, Esq., the representative of the borough; S. Amory, Esq., of London; F. Hale, Esq., George Coles, Esq., A. Brewin, Esq., H. Dumford, Esq., John Barne, Esq., J. Hopgood, Esq., T. Rendell, Esq., F. O. Patch, Esq., A. C. Sharland, Esq.; H. U. Janson, Esq. and R. Parker, Esq., of Exeter; and Messrs. Jackson and Davey, the well known mesmeric lecturers.

From this period the attacks which had at first so distressed me were lessened, and they gradually yielded as facts were produced and accumulated evidence was given. My operations were not confined to weak, enervated persons. By far the greater number were muscular agricultnral labourers, who, in the west of England, particularly in Devonshire, from sudden changes of temperature are subject to severe rheumatic pains. These are greatly modified and frequently disappear after a few applications of mesmeric passes.

As we all possess more or less of this sanitary influence, every head of a family ought to be a mesmerist, more especially in his own circle: every mother ought to operate on her child. It is time for females to divest themselves of the idea that they have no power or force. As a proof to the contrary I may quote the lady of Dr. Whateley, Archbishop of Dublin, who cured a female of blindness after mesmerising her almost daily for three years (*Zoist*, No. xxv., p. 81). Miss Wallace (*Zoist*, Nos. iii., iv., vi., vii.), and Miss Martineau (*Zoist*, Vol. viii., p. 300), have also furnished proofs of their moral courage, and are examples worthy of all imitation. The latter lady has been ill treated for an act of mercy to her cow (*Zoist*, Vol. viii., pp. 334-5). I have witnessed similar proofs of the power of mesmerism on quadrupeds and birds: in fact I have been the operator.

It is highly satisfactory to witness the increased desire manifested by the clergy and ministers of religion of every denomination to become acquainted with our important truths for the purpose of extending their own usefulness to their poor parishioners. What on earth can be more beautiful than witnessing a minister of the gospel operating on a poor, suffering fellow-creature, and, after affording quietude and ease, directing the attention of the recipient of the blessing to a higher power. For, as the will and desire to do good is necessary, it may be more beneficial from the hands of men who are bound to be holy and whose whole life should be one of mercy and charity. Numbers of the preachers of the gospel have become subscribers to this work. A humble operator—one to "fortune and to fame unknown," as the *Medical Times* styles me in impotent derision—I am delighted to be placed in the rear of so many good and holy persons as are daily engaged in operating and diffusing a knowledge of this God-like power.

Works of this character should lie on the shelf of every family, however humble, as well as in the library of the affluent. It is very satisfactory to find the faculty are putting their houses in order, and preparing for a change: they only require, as is required in some other cases, a pressure from without. One of the leading physicians in the metropolis has given instructions to his nurses to shampoo his patients after the manner of mesmerists. They are thus preparing for some great change. The public press to this time has not done justice to the science; but has lately, however, shewn a disposition to quit the stronghold of scepticism. Within a few weeks there have been unmistakable evidences of a great change about being effected. Let those gentlemen who cater for the public, occasionally accompany the mesmerist to the abode of misery and disease and view the effects produced. Let them hear the afflicted relate how pain is driven from various parts of the body until it disappears at the toes or fingers: and let him view the great relief afforded to the disordered brain. It here appears in its plenitude of power and beauty. The phrenzied brain may be subdued, and the mind of an insane person brought to its original state, notwithstanding Dr. Conolly's contempt for mesmerism.*

* Many cures of insanity are recorded in *The Zoist*, and Dr. Kean reports that in the Lunatic Asylum at Berhampore 74 pa-

The treatment of the insane, the most unfortunate of God's creatures, has been too frequently very defective.

With those positive facts, are we not justified in calling upon the medical profession to enquire into the application of this mighty power, instead of abusing and insulting those who are willing to confer a boon and a benefit upon suffering humanity. We hear of the power of the press. Let the gentlemen belonging to it at once enter into the enquiry, and they will soon, very soon, discover whether this power is of Satanic origin, as has occasionally been promulgated from the pulpit. As to the proof of its efficacy in preventing the pain of the most terrible surgical operations, as well as in cases of insanity and many other diseases, let the most fastidious read the statements as forwarded by Dr. Esdaile from

tients were mesmerised, and 64 of these discharged in the years 1847-8, apparently cured; *Zoist*, Vol. VII., p. 362. At p. 136 we read, "Dr. Kean informs us, *that since the employment of mesmerism almost all difficulty in the management of the patients has vanished.* Formerly, there were always a number of noisy and violent patients, and a good many who slept neither day nor night, for weeks together, in spite of every remedial measure. *Now the whole are as orderly and quiet as an equal number of persons in any other house, and all enjoy natural rest. So great is the change that Dr. Kean says he could, with additional burkundauzes, as easily manage* 500 *as* 50 *patients!*"

the establishments at Calcutta that are in the hands of the Government; one tumour being taken from a man's body weighing above a hundred, and many almost a hundred, pounds, whilst the patients were in a mesmeric sleep, without their feeling the slightest pain. The time is approaching when justice will be done to those who have been injured—more particularly to Dr. Elliotson. Yes, posterity will appreciate his merits and will regret that Englishmen should have abandoned themselves so far as to heap calumny, abuse, and insult, and inflict immense pecuniary injury, on this great man.

It was intended that this work should contain about one hundred and fifty cases, but it might have extended to above three or even four hundred statements. I shall be sufficiently repaid, if, by the publicity of those cases, a few individuals step forward and take Drs. Elliotson and Ashburner as their guiding stars. For my own part I may confidently state, after my long course of well intended labours, that I believe the subject is one of incalculable importance, and that these efforts of mine have had their own reward; and that the number of cases in which I have been enabled to administer relief is such as fully to warrant my asking the attention of all to the means employed. If it be the fact that relief from pain is thus obtained, strength restored to the withered limb, and repose procured for those who need it, surely this of itself is enough to recommend to your favour a process so simple that any one who may think fit can exercise it for the benefit of those who are deficient in what he possesses, and thus, at no cost beyond his time, become an instrument of blessing to those around him. If these results be, as I maintain they are, the consequences of the application of this principle, it is but of little importance whether, in our present state of knowledge, it admit of a philosophical explanation or not.

The public must determine whether the facts in my little book are of more weight than the opinions of the medical world which is still quite ignorant of mesmerism. These opinions I will present to my readers as taken from the records of what Mr. Janson truly calls "the wonderful *Zoist*," and which is the most important book of the present age.

THOMAS CAPERN.

9, Bedford Street, Bedford Square,
February 1, 1851.

Lancet.

"Careful investigation and consideration of all the experiments have convinced us that the phenomena are not real, and that animal magnetism is a *delusion*. We shall, therefore, lose no opportunity of extirpating an error, which in its *nature*, *application*, and *consequences*, is PERNICIOUS."—Sept. 8th, 1838.

"*Life, Adventures, and Death* of Animal Magnetism."—*Cover of Lancet*, Sept. 8th, 1838.

Mr. Wakley's own experiments, he declares in this number, "utterly destroyed the facts adduced in this country in favour of that *delusion*," p. 356.

"The science of mesmerism dares no longer affront the common sense of the medical profession, or dares to shew its face after the last exposure."—Sept. 15th, 1838.

"We cannot insert any communication in support of the EXTRAVAGANT HUMBUG of animal magnetism."—Dec. 8th, 1838.

"Mesmerism is too *gross a humbug* to admit of any farther serious notice. We regard *its abettors* as *quacks and impostors*. They ought to be *hooted out of professional society*.—Any practitioner who sends a patient afflicted with *any* disease to consult a mesmeric quack, ought to be without patients for the rest of his days."—Oct. 29, 1842.

"If there are still any doubters as to mesmerism being a *fraud*, we advise them to peruse this pamphlet (Dr. Forbes's Illustrations of Modern Mesmerism). It certainly is a prickly rod for one of those classes of modern *quacks*." 1844.

"Look at the chosen audience and instruments of this mesmeric leader (Dr. Elliotson). Does he himself treat the harlotry which he dares to call science with any respect? Let the profession consider his allies and assistants, taken from the pert folly of the nobility, the weakest among the literary people, high and low ladies, *quack clergymen*, itinerant lecturers and exhibiting buffoons."—July 4, 1846.

"We cannot publish any papers on the subject of such an *odious fraud* as mesmerism."—July 22, 1848.

"If we read the signs of the times aright, we believe that one effect of the protrusion of these *audacious quackeries* (mesmerism, &c.) into the face of day, will be to unite the profession strongly against those who trade in them, or those medical persons and others who keep the traders in countenance."—April 20, p. 369.

Medico-Chirurgical Review.

"The mesmero-mania has nearly dwindled, in the metropolis, into anile fatuity; but lingers in some of the provinces with the *gobe-mouches* and chaw-bacons, who, after gulping down a pound of fat pork, would, with well-greased gullets, swallow such a lot of mesmeric mummery as would choke an alligator or a boa constrictor."

"We laugh at the folly, we pity the madness, of the mesmerists. Many of them are neither better nor worse than arrant charlatans—more are weak dupes of knaves or of themselves—and a few are sincere, *high-principled fanatics*, led away by a love of the extravagant and marvellous, and trying very earnestly, but with small success, to hold the eel of philosophy by the tail."

"For our parts, we view mesmerism as a ludicrous, *if not a mischievous delusion*, and, without regard to persons, *it should be laughed at and put down*."—*Dr. James Johnson*, April 1, 1843.

British and Foreign Medical Review.

"Nevertheless there is comfort. The world is round, saith the proverb, and all things come to an end. *Pass a few short months and the delusion stands exposed; the actors are declared to be deceivers or deceived; the facts so lately boasted of are trampled upon with contempt, and the doctrines built upon them are laughed to scorn.* The fashionable crowd flock to a new *prima donna* or to a watering-place doctor; and the half-converted physicians and surgeons never mention the subject more; for, although the folly will rise again, it will scarcely be in their time."

"We beheld, always with astonishment, sometimes with concern, and sometimes with contempt, the credulity, real or pretended, of the magnetizers. We observed, with some little disgust, here and there a practitioner willing to become the *provincial* wonder, and only restrained by his prudence from declaring what a mixture of *ignorance and cupidity* prepared him to assert and to do. But above all, we lamented to see the *great delusion* supported by one of the ablest physicians of this country, filling the most important chair in the largest medical school of the kingdom."

"Considering the high sanction which even a temporary belief in the powers of animal magnetism has obtained in this country, we look upon its recent rise and progress, and ITS ABRUPT AND SHAMEFUL FALL, as powerfully calculated to degrade a profession which is certainly, for other reasons, not rising in public estimation."

"To devote an article to the consideration of animal magnetism, *now that the English practitioners are one and all ashamed of its name*, would be a work of supererogation, if the delusion, unabashed, were not yet parading itself over some parts of the continent; (!)—and if its return to these shores, and to our own hospitals and colleges, at any future period, were quite out of the question. But if we can quicken *its decline* where it now reigns in the hearts of nervous proselytes and *dreaming physicians*, or can assist in forming a barrier against a probable revisitation of it, we shall not think the otherwise more than due attention we have given to the wild productions which treat of it, entirely thrown away."—*Drs. Forbes and Conolly*, April, 1839.

On Nov. 30, 1848, Dr. Conolly advertised in the newspapers that he rejected mesmerism. See *Zoist*, No. XXIV., p. 369.

London Medical Gazette.

"The Journal *(The Zoist)* only finds countenance among the class of *impostors* who record their own doings in it."—April 12, 1845.

"It is with mingled regret and pity that we now receive Dr. Herbert Mayo's admission of the so called *truth* of mesmerism. We cannot but feel a degree of doubt of the vigour of a mind once accustomed to the serious investigation of the sciences of physiology and pathology. We cannot but lament that the author should be content to throw away a well-earned reputation by the advancing of the claims of such things as mesmerism and hydropathy."—Oct. 12, 1849.

Medical Times.

"If the same amount of deliberate imposture cannot be brought home to the mesmerists of our time, it is not owing to there being a greater allowance of truth in their system, but because self-deception exists among the professors to a greater extent, and probably because the dupes being the very *élite* of human weakness yield their belief without the trouble of much lying."—April 13, 1850.

"As to the cure of diseases by mesmerism, it is contemptible." —April 27, 1850.

"We shall not, therefore, allow this heresy [mesmerism] still to be propagated under the pretext of its having any pretension even to the name of a science. *Judex damnatur cum nocens absolvitur;* we shall bruise the head of the serpent, and leave it to trail its wounded length, hissing but harmless, along its tortuous paths for the remainder of its days."—Aug. 31, 1850.

"The Mesmeric Cases reported by Mr. Capern, Mr. Mott, Mr. Parker, and Mr. Tubbs, (gentlemen whose euphonious names are at present, professionally, "to fortune and to fame unknown,") may be summarily dismissed. They remind us only of the significant couplet in the poem of Dr. Syntax, where the bookseller, shaking his head at the manuscript of the poor traveller, reminds him—

"'We can get tours—don't make wry faces—
From those who never saw the places.'

Which may be thus travestied:—

"We can get *facts*—don't make wry faces—
From those who never saw the *cases!*"

August 31, 1850.

The Institute, a medical Journal, belonging to Mr. Martin, Surgeon, Reigate.

". . . That *mean and contemptible delusion*—MESMERISM—*Refuted, exposed*, and only saved from utter annihilation by the tenacity with which one individual, and he, unfortunately, a medical man, clings to it."—Nov. 9, 1850.

"All its pretended facts were scattered to the winds by the application of a little common sense, and a few experiments made by Mr. Wakley. . . Is it possible to receive the testimony of persons once so exposed, so convicted of either incompetency to deal with physical science, or unfaithfulness to the holy cause of truth and honesty? We think not, and therefore reject as fabulous the alleged power of 'manipulations' and 'passes,' to render any one insensible to the pain of surgical operations. We have now several definite physical agents, ether, chloroform, &c., to effect this purpose completely; but the influence of these anæsthetics gives no support to the power of mesmerism."—Nov. 30, 1850.

Weekly Dispatch.

"That mesmerism is at best a delusion, is clear, for it is adopted by no respectable practitioner of the medical profession, the only man of respectability that has adopted it being on this subject supposed by his brethren to be insane. It is a monomania, that has caused him the loss of his extensive practice, and it has converted the esteem of his friends into pity. The North London Hospital shewed its good sense by compelling this unfortunate physician to cease to lecture, and to vacate his offices. No public establishment has adopted mesmerism. It has not appeared in our colleges, halls, universities, or other places of science of any description; or where it has appeared, it has only been either to die a natural death, or to be scouted at by all honest and respectable people."—May 14, 1844.*

* I quote the *Dispatch* to shew the state of the medical profession. But it is a duty to quote a paragraph which appeared on the 12th of January, 1851, the paper being now conducted by better brains. "Dr. Elliotson is the ablest of the professors of

Mr. Turner, of Manchester, called for the imposition of pains and penalties. He says, "We ought to demand at once that Government interfere most imperiously to protect the morals of the people, by putting an instrument of such weight and power within proper hands only to execute it." "I would have the legislative measure without waiting for any investigation into the extravagances of mesmerism."—See *Zoist*, Vol. ii., p. 280.

College of Physicians.

"Do not QUACKS hunt out the vices or infirmities of mankind to turn them to profit, some selecting one and some another for their purpose? Among quacks, the IMPOSTORS called MESMERISTS, are in my opinion the especial FAVOURITES of those, both male and female, in whom the SEXUAL PASSIONS BURN STRONGLY, either in secret or notoriously. DECENCY FORBIDS ME TO BE MORE EXPLICIT.

"From these and similar ARTIFICES, the physician should be carefully removed and guarded: and this can hardly be accomplished except by a sound education, which will teach him to thoroughly abhor all DECEIT AND TRICK."—*Harveian Oration, delivered by* DR. F. HAWKINS BEFORE THE LONDON COLLEGE OF PHYSICIANS, June 24, 1848.

"Of those forward female creatures who busy themselves in-

mesmerism, and there is no doubt whatever that the power may be directed to the cure of diseases. A hospital has been opened in the vicinity of Bedford-row for the cure of diseases by mesmerism. The palsy is one of the ailments to which this remedy has been applied with success, but it is also extensively practised in the East Indies for producing insensiblity to pain while operations are carried on."

cessantly with every strange practice in medicine, surgery, and midwifery, and clamour in public without any modesty for this or that man-midwife who happens to be their delight, contrary to the teaching, the morals, and the innocence of Harvey,—of this or that duke, earl, senator, knight, who trust their wives or daughters to these *indecent* MESMERIC *or obstetric women—of mesmeric bishops, of arch-mesmeric arch-bishops*,—allow me for this one day, while I am among my brother doctors, to hold my tongue out of sheer *disgust*, *out of modesty*, *out of* MY REVERENCE FOR RELIGION !"

" *Get out of the way you modern patrons, you homœopathists, you hydropathists, you visionaries, you* MESMERISTS. Your ways, your nature, disqualify you for patronizing in conjunction with that pure old English breed of the nobleman and the physician."

" Do, pray, let the absurdities, the presumption, the indecencies, with which you have so long oppressed and almost extinguished our divine art, be banished for ever into utter darkness and silence by this adjuration at least."

" To all who cultivate genuine medicine daily, diligently, and most laboriously, who try to preserve their good feelings and the excellence of their nature, purity, and morals—to all who prefer living in honest poverty to growing rich by the systematic quackeries of homœopathy, hydropathy, and MESMERISM—to all these respectable fellows of the College, though humble in ambition and pocket, let us return due thanks solemnly in obedience to Harvey, as to our benefactors."—Dr. J. A. WILSON's *Harveian Oration, delivered in* 1850, *before the London College of Physicians.*

Dr. Elliotson in vain attempted to obtain redress from the

College. The President, Dr. Paris, took no notice of a polite note: and, on Dr. Elliotson writing again at the end of three months, had recourse to a silly and mean evasion by replying that he could not enter into a controversy respecting mesmerism. On which Dr. Elliotson wrote :—

"Dr. Elliotson presents his compliments to the President of the Royal College of Physicians of London, and begs to remark that he did not request the President's attention to passages of Dr. Francis Hawkins's Oration relating to *mesmerism*, or of a controversial character, for there are none such; but to passages relating to *mesmerists*, of whom he, a Fellow of the College, has for ten years openly been one—passages stigmatizing mesmerists as quacks and impostors and the especial favourites of both males and females whose sexual passions are secretly or notoriously violent; respecting which point Dr. Hawkins declared that decency forbad him to say more.

"Conduit Street, Nov. 17, 1848."

Dr. E. adds :—"To this I have received no reply. The matter is now for posterity."—*Zoist*, Vol. vi., p. 399.

University College.

"Resolved, That the hospital committee be instructed to take such steps as they shall deem most advisable to prevent the practice of mesmerism or animal magnetism in future within this hospital." —*Minutes of the Council*, Dec. 27, 1838.

Dr. Elliotson's colleague, Mr. Liston, asked if he had not disappeared: maintained that the Okeys were trained: that a person would go to sleep if you ——— in his face: and declared that he would resign his professorship if that tom-fool, Elliotson, returned to the hospital. Another colleague, Dr. A. T. Thompson, said, "Thank God, we have got rid of him;" and boasted to his class, that, although mesmeric cases were to be seen in the same ward with his own patients, he had never looked at one of them. We remember that this professor was hissed by his students for speaking ill of Dr. Elliotson after he had resigned.—*Zoist*, Vol. ii. p. 283.

The Royal Medical and Chirurgical Society,

After having had read to them the details of an amputation which was performed unconsciously in the mesmeric state, were violent and resolved at the next meeting to erase from their minutes all trace of such a paper having been read. The foremost of those antimesmerists who were amusing at the two meetings were Sir B. Brodie, Mr. Liston, Mr. Bransby Cooper, Dr. Copland, Mr. Cæsar Hawkins, Dr. Marshall Hall, Dr. James Johnson, and Dr. George Gregory."—See Dr. Elliotson's remarkable pamphlet, called "Numerous Surgical Operations without Pain in the Mesmeric State; with Remarks upon the Opposition of many Members of the Royal Medical and Chirurgical Society and others to the reception of the inestimable blessings of Mesmerism."

Sir B. Brodie and Dr. Chambers, like Dr. James Johnson, have repeatedly said that they would not go to see a case of mesmerism, and, if they saw one, would not believe what they saw.

CURATIVE POWERS OF MESMERISM.

SECTION I.

RHEUMATISM.

1. J. Fowler.—In reply to an enquiry as to my recollection of the case of J. Fowler, of Home Farm, in this parish, I well remember that about two years ago he called upon me to inform me that for several years before he had been seriously afflicted with rheumatic pains in his arm and shoulder, that began soon after his falling from his father's hay-loft. He also said that he had had recourse to various means of relief without any effect whatever: but, on calling on Mr. Capern that morning, and after having had Mr. C.'s hand applied to the parts where he had experienced so much pain, he enjoyed immediate relief,—so much so that he could raise his hand above his head without the least inconvenience,—a thing he had not been able to do for several years before. He then threw his hands up over his head, declaring that for years before he had not been able to raise them above his ears.

I have taken great interest in the exercise of Mr. C.'s mesmeric powers, having had scores of instances before me of the extraordinary relief afforded by him. I have also taken some trouble to investigate very minutely the characters of many of those who have assured me of the benefit they have received. The result has been very satisfactory: insomuch, that I deem them worthy of belief in every particular which they declared to be true in my presence.

I shall only add that it is with very great regret I hear that Mr. Capern is about leaving us to take up his residence in London. His absence will be felt greatly by his poorer neighbours; while his excellent conduct and behaviour, his kindness and his usefulness, have most deservedly obtained for him the respect of all classes inhabiting his native town.

(Signed) GEORGE COLES,
Magistrate for the Borough of Tiverton.

Tiverton, Sept. 17, 1850.

2. JOHN CROOTE, mason, aged 49 years, caught a chill through working in an oven, and was ill for nearly five years: for two years and a quarter of the time he was under treatment by the medical officers of the Exeter Hospital, both as an in and out patient; he was an in-patient twelve months, when, finding that he was no better, he left the institution and returned to Tiverton. On his return home, he felt some improvement, which induced him to resume work: but he was unable to complete even one week of labour. On the sixth day he suddenly became so ill that he was obliged to be assisted home by two of his fellow-workmen. With the exception of not quite six days on this occasion, he was unable to do a stroke of work during the whole period of his illness. Becoming worse and worse, he placed

himself under the care of the parish doctor; but there was no improvement. After an absence of about four or five months he returned to the hospital at Exeter. While there, he was in a most pitiable state; he suffered extreme pain over almost the whole body; even with crutches he was unable to move about, or go up and down stairs without assistance. He lost strength and flesh, became extremely weak and emaciated, and had little or no appetite. Despairing of ever getting better, he at length returned home. His neighbours all thought that he was a dying man, and that in a few weeks he would be in his grave. A person with whom he had formerly worked had several times invited him down to his house, which is situated at some distance from his own residence. After having several times refused, he at length, with the assistance of two men, managed to make his way down to him. He strongly advised him to apply to Mr. Capern, of whose mesmeric cures he had never heard before. Mr. Capern, happening just then to pass the door, was invited to come in, and at once commenced the usual manipulations. Almost at the very first pass the patient felt a strong sensation of warmth, and in a few minutes he was almost entirely free from pain; at the conclusion of the operation he walked home without assistance in perfect ease, carrying his crutches over his shoulders. On his way homewards he felt somewhat drowsy, and, on his reaching his own house, felt so irresistible an inclination to sleep that he threw himself upon the bed and slept uninterruptedly for sixteen hours. During the eight weeks previous he had not, he declares, had an hour's sleep. His wife was so alarmed at the length of his nap that she called in her neighbours, one after the other, to try to awake him; but their efforts were in vain. He awoke spontaneously, greatly refreshed and quite free from pain. The operation was repeated, but not every day, for ten or twelve weeks. His recovery was rapid: in eleven weeks he increased in weight forty-two pounds. In five or six weeks after his first application to Mr. Capern he was able to do a little work: in ten or twelve weeks he was in full employ, and not many weeks afterwards he was not only able to do a good day's work, but to walk five miles to his labour and five miles back every day in the depth of winter, and over one of the worst roads in the county. He is now as strong and well as he ever was in his life. It is nearly three years since his cure was effected. He was told at Exeter by the surgeons of the hospital that he would never be able to do a day's work again. During the last eight weeks of the two years and a quarter that he was a patient of the hospital he drank sixteen quarts of very nauseous oil.

About two months since, in November, 1849, he being in Exeter on business, took the opportunity of paying a visit to the hospital, to see the surgeon under whose care he had been when in the institution, and some of the attendants. The alteration in his appearance was so great that those who saw him could scarcely believe that he was the same person.

J. Croote.

Mem.—During the treatment of this case, the patient experienced at one time considerable pain in the leg.

By way of experiment, I made the passes through an iron of two-pounds weight, which I held with my left hand over the seat of the pain at the distance of two or three inches. Before this, the passes had invariably caused a strong sensation of warmth, but on this occasion intense cold was felt in the part immediately under the iron, extending quite through the limb, and diffused over a space exactly corresponding to the size of the weight. Nothing that the patient could do produced any warmth in the part; he sometimes stood holding the limb so close to the fire as to singe his clothes, without the sensation of cold being in the least diminished; and the passes which I made were equally ineffective. After this had continued two or three weeks, I one day tried the experiment of making the passes through a heated body,—a piece of marble, about an inch and a half thick, held over the part: and the sense of cold instantaneously disappeared. Mr. Croote appears to be extremely susceptible to the influence of metals and crystals. A piece of silver being drawn a few days since over the hand in the manner mentioned by Reichenbach, he felt very considerable pain down the arm, particularly at the elbow joint. The same result took place when a piece of rock crystal was substituted for the silver. A few passes removed the pain.

THOMAS CAPERN.

3. SAMUEL CHUDLEIGH, aged 68 years, parish of Coleford, near Crediton, was suddenly seized five years ago with pains all over his body. On the second day he was compelled to go to bed. The doctor of the

union attended him, but without any benefit. In a fortnight, being much worse, he was removed to the Exeter Hospital. While there he continued getting worse, and at the end of a fortnight requested to be sent home, as he thought he should die if he staid any longer. He was conveyed home with great difficulty, and was then confined to his bed for a year and ten months. He was again attended by the union surgeon, who, however, did him no good: indeed, often told him that his case was hopeless. During this time he suffered great pain: his legs and arms became contracted, and he felt as if they were chained together; and, the disease attacking his eyes, he lost the sight of the right. At the end of that time, however, he improved a little, and was able to leave his bed. His legs still remained contracted, and he was quite unable to move without crutches. In that state he remained for three years more, when his son, who resided at Tiverton, advised him to apply to Mr. Capern. He accordingly came to Tiverton, a distance of sixteen miles, and on the 26th February Mr. Capern mesmerised him for the first time. He felt considerable warmth in the limbs, and slept better that night than he had ever done since he was first ill. After six mesmerisations he was able to walk without crutches, and go up and down stairs in the ordinary manner, which he had not been able to do for five years. He now sleeps well and feels no pain, and, though the limbs are still contracted, he is able to walk without any inconvenience, and expresses great gratitude to Mr. Capern for the good he has done him.

A remarkable fact connected with this patient is that

he has been practising "mesmerism" unconsciously from the day of his birth up to the present time. A popular superstition exists in Devonshire that every seventh son possesses the power of curing disease by the simple application of the hand. So firmly is this believed that persons were waiting anxiously for his birth in order to be touched by the new-born infant, should it be a boy, for the cure of their diseases. This power he exercises every Sunday only—the day of the week on which he was born. At the time of operating he mentally repeats what is believed to be a portion of Scripture; but on this point he was not communicative. He commences by making seven passes over the diseased part precisely in the mode adopted by mesmerists, decreasing the number of passes every Sunday by one until he comes to the last; always, however, taking the same time in making each lesser number of passes that he had previously taken in making the seven, so that the one pass on the seventh Sunday occupies as much time as the seven passes did on the first. Should the cure, however, not have been effected at the termination of the seventh Sunday when the last pass is made, a second course is commenced the Sunday following, seven passes being again made and the number decreased each Sunday as before. During his stay in Tiverton, whilst under Mr. Capern, he was visited every Sunday by persons suffering from scrofula, on whom he operated in his usual manner. Two of these, Mr. Upton, of Bickleigh, and Mr. Clarke, declare themselves much benefitted, and I allude to their cases as they came under my own observation. His father, being also a seventh son, practised the cure of disease in the same manner: and my patient was believed to possess extraordinary powers of healing because he was the seventh son of a seventh son.

In addition to his operation, a sixpence or other piece of silver is sewn into a small bag, and that again into another, and worn round the operator's neck during the last of the seven weeks. It is then given to the patient, who wears it for the next seven weeks, and it is afterwards deposited in a box to be carefully preserved from wet or the touch of a needle. Should this not be carefully attended to, the disease will return; and he states that he has known cases where, the above precautions not being properly attended to, the disease has returned.

4. Thomas Winsborough, agricultural labourer, Barton, Tiverton, aged 76, states that about five years since he caught a chill in consequence of frequent exposure to rain and standing on wet ground. At length he had severe rheumatism; so severe as at times to prevent him from labouring for three successive months, and he was frequently compelled either to walk about the room or sit by the fire whole nights together in the midst of winter. Such was his condition from the intense pain at his advanced age that he looked forward to a total incapacity of labour or exertion, and which he believes, but for Mr. Capern's kindness, would have been the result. It is now nearly three years since he was induced to name it to Mr. Capern, who consented to operate upon him. The first time the passes were made on him by the palm of the hand over the affected

parts he experienced less pain. He attended daily, with advantage, for one week, and afterwards less frequently for a fortnight. At the end of that period he was completely cured; and he has had no return of the pain since.

Tiverton, December, 1850.

5. Elizabeth Kerslake, wife of John Kerslake, of Sampford Peverell, aged 35. Had for five years a very severe attack of rheumatism in the right shoulder down the side and leg. At times she could not move the arms for months together. The pains frequently moved from the arm to the hip and leg. The last attack she experienced was nine months since. It was with difficulty she could walk across the room. For eight weeks previous to applying to Mr. Capern (about seven months since), she tried a variety of means which were recommended by her friends, and had medical advice, but received no benefit. She was operated upon on a Tuesday for the first time, but felt no particular sensation. The operation was repeated on the following Saturday, after which she felt improved. She attended four times afterwards, and has felt no pain since.

6. John Lentall, aged 23 years, in the employ of Messrs. Davey and Cosway, limeburners, was attacked about three months since with acute pains in the right side of the head and jaw. His nights were restless. He applied to a druggist who tried various remedies. He used embrocations, baths, and herbs, but without experiencing any alleviation of the pain. At length a

fellow workman of his, who had been relieved by Mr. Capern when suffering, recommended his being mesmerised. On Friday, the 22nd of March, he attended at Mr. C.'s house, and a few minutes after Mr. Capern's hands had been passed over the side of the head he felt considerably relieved. On the 23rd he was again operated on with further improvement. He attended again on the 25th, and now states he has had no pain or inconvenience since.

7. John Gill, aged 35, drainer, Ash Village, near Tiverton, in the employ of John Heathcoat, Esq., suffered severe pains in the leg, from the knee to the foot, for three years. It was supposed to be a rheumatic affection, occasioned by frequent working in water. Frequently the pains were so excessive that he felt relief only by walking the room at night. The pains generally were more severe between the hours of ten and twelve, p.m., and continued till about five in the morning. He applied to a surgeon and a druggist in Tiverton without benefit. He then applied to Mr. Capern, and after the first mesmerisation a sensation of heat was produced. He attended five times, and was operated upon from ten to twelve minutes each time. He is now quite well and free from pain.

8. Ann Martin, widow, Frog Street, Tiverton, aged 53, suffered between two and three years from rheumatic affection in the right leg, and more particularly in the knee. The swelling was so great and painful as at times to deprive her of all rest. She applied

various liniments and oils without effect. The swelling could not be reduced by the ordinary means. She applied to Mr. Capern, and after the first sitting she walked with more ease than she had done during the above mentioned period; and after three sittings she was completely cured, and has had no return of the pain or swelling in the knee from that time. This took place about two years since.

April 4th, 1850.

9. Copy of a written statement, received from Daniel Pardue, a stranger, who, whilst attending Tiverton fair, September 29th, 1847, was seized with a rheumatic attack:—

"Tiverton, Dec. 3rd, 1847.

"This is to certify that I had the rheumatic pains so bad in my arms that I could not move them without help until visited by Mr. Thomas Capern, who very kindly tried the experiment of mesmerism with success. The first time I nearly fainted. Since then he has visited me daily, and I am now enabled to use my arms.

"DANIEL PARDUE."

Mem.—Daniel Pardue was attended by a surgeon, previously to being operated upon.

10. Copy of a statement received from James Summers, of Sampford Peverell, yeoman.

"Sampford Peverell, Oct. 28th, 1849.

"I, James Summers, hereby certify that I was suffering a continuous and acute pain in the hip joint and legs for upwards of five weeks, so that at times I was not able to walk across the room. On application to my medical attendant, he stated that probably it originated from a chill, and that he believed it to be rheumatic affection. From him I took many doses of medicine, and was bled; but, receiving no benefit, I applied to Mr. Capern of Tiverton, who with pleasure instantly mesmerised the affected side. A comfortable heat was produced, and instantaneous relief afforded. I was astonished at the ease I experienced on my return to Sampford. A short time afterwards, I again stated to Mr. Capern that I had sensations of pain, although much less severe than formerly. My friend again operated upon me, which caused an entire cessation of pain; and I have been wholly free from that complaint ever since, and can now perform any kind of labour without inconvenience.

"James Summers."

11. Statement from Maria Peaster.

"I, Maria Peaster, of Leat Street, Tiverton, certify that I was suffering severe pains in the head for three successive years; and the last year of that time I was frequently incapable of labour. I was advised by many persons to apply to Mr. Capern, and, although faithless of the power, I did so, and was entirely cured at the first sitting. This was twelve months since; and I have experienced no pain from that time.

"Maria Peaster.

"Tiverton, Nov. 7th, 1849."

12. JOHN FERRIS, yeoman, Tiverton, aged 64, was a great sufferer from rheumatism for upwards of twenty years: during which time he was often confined to his bed and entirely disabled from work; and was occasionally so crippled as to be unable for weeks together to cut his food. The pain first appeared in the groin, and was often extremely violent, especially at night. He had constant lameness, and for many years was unable to get over a stile in the usual manner, but was accustomed to seat himself upon the rail, swing himself round, and then deposit his legs upon the opposite side. After a time the pain flew to the back. At or about the period of its shifting, he was confined to his bed for a fortnight, and treated medically, with but little relief; nevertheless, in process of time, he became better, and was able to follow his usual occupation. The seat of pain then shifted to the collar bone. The pain was excruciating, and he had little or no sleep in consequence of his sufferings. He consulted several medical men at various times; and, besides the medicines which they prescribed, had recourse to a variety of remedies recommended to him by others; but without benefit. He had never heard of mesmerism till he came in one day, between two and three years ago, to see Mr. Capern on business. Not finding Mr. C. at home, he sat down in the kitchen to await his return. In the interval, another person came in who entered into conversation with Mr. Capern's servant upon the subject of mesmerism and her master's mesmeric cures. This excited the curiosity of Mr. Ferris and induced him to enquire what this wonderful mesmerism was; and, after having seen the

other person who had come in completely relieved by a few passes from Mr. Capern, he willingly submitted himself to the operation, and in ten minutes or a quarter of an hour was entirely free from pain. He has remained so, with few exceptions, ever since. Occasionally he feels some slight pains, principally in the groin; but a few passes from Mr. Capern never fail to afford complete relief. Between two and three months ago he suffered somewhat more severely in the same part, and applied to Mr. Capern, who relieved him effectually in a few minutes.

13. James Gill, Tiverton, weaver, in the employ of Mr. Cosway, was afflicted with rheumatism in the left arm and shoulder for three months. He suffered much pain, was unable to put on his coat without assistance, and could do but little work. After Mr. Capern had operated upon him two or three times, the pain entirely left him. He has not complained since. The cure was effected about two years and a half ago.

14. Copy of a letter from Mr. Thomas Stevens, Landside Farm, Sampford Peverell, Yeoman.

"This is to certify that after being a great sufferer, upwards of nine months, in my shoulder, from the fall of a horse, I was persuaded to apply to Mr. Capern, Peters Street, Tiverton, to be mesmerised: and so I did, and within a fortnight, I was perfectly sound.

"Yours, &c.,

"Thomas Stevens.

"Sampford Peverell, Oct. 5th, 1848."

15. I, NICHOLAS SEARLES, agricultural labourer, of Bampton, do hereby certify that I have suffered very severe pains for seven years past; and for the last three years have been incapable of performing any kind of labour; and at times I was so weakened and suffered so much pain as to be incapable of raising myself from my chair. I was for the greater part of the time under the care of a surgeon, who, after trying various means, assured me that medicine would not benefit me and advised me to desist from taking any. Being recommended to apply to Mr. Capern, I was induced to do so, who kindly consented, and, after making a few passes over my back and knee which was the principal seat of the pain, I immediately experienced relief, and felt more ease than I had for several years. I again called on Mr. C. at the end of a fortnight, when I was further relieved: in fact, I was enabled to walk from Bampton to Cullompton, a distance of thirteen miles, with comparative ease and comfort; which I should not have attempted but for the exertions of my friend. On the Friday following, I again walked from Cullompton to Bampton, and was again operated upon. From that time I have been enabled to work on the farm with ease to myself and satisfaction to my employer.

16. WILLIAM HAWKINS, agricultural labourer, of Cadeleigh. In answer to a letter from Mr. Capern, the following is the reply:—"Sir, I was ill nearly two years; lost many days' work. I came once to you: I

lost the pain immediately, and have not felt it since. The pains were in the knee and arm.

"WILLIAM HAWKINS."

17. ROBERT HOLE, labourer, Sharlands Court, suffered rheumatic pains in the arm and shoulder for six weeks, during which time he was unable to work or even use his arm at all. He had surgeons attending him during that time, who continually applied blisters; but he received no benefit therefrom. The first time he saw Mr. Capern, he had four blisters on. After a few passes were made, he felt great relief. This was on a Friday; and, on the following Monday, he was able to resume his labour, and he is now as well as ever.

18. MRS. TURNER, wife of Mr. John Turner, schoolmaster, aged 63, states as follows:—"I was troubled with rheumatic pains for five years: I could not walk about the house without crutches. I applied to Mr. Capern, at the request of my neighbours, and after the passes had been made five times I was quite recovered."

19. WILLIAM GILL, agricultural labourer, in the employ of Thomas B. Talley, Esq., was for ten or twelve years a great sufferer from rheumatism: the pain was sometimes so severe as to keep him from work for days together. He was in great pain, and scarcely able to walk, when he first applied to Mr. Capern. By a few passes he was completely relieved, and walked

home with perfect ease, and quite free from pain. About six months afterwards he had a severe attack. He was engaged in removing manure, but was obliged to have a man to load his cart for him, as he was unable to handle the shovel himself. Mr. Capern happened to meet him while he was in this state, again operated upon him, and afforded him complete relief. He occasionally suffers slightly when the weather is unfavourable; but the pain on these occasions is not to be compared with what he formerly felt.

20. ——— ————, aged 50, was for four or five years subject to severe and sudden attacks of rheumatic pains; they usually lasted some hours, and were sometimes so violent that he was hardly able to get up and down stairs. About two years ago he was mesmerised by Mr. Capern, and has remained quite well ever since.

21. James Webber, Bampton Down, agricultural labourer, aged 52, severe rheumatism first in the back, then over the whole body, for twenty-two years. The first attack lasted fifteen months, during the whole of which time he was entirely incapable of labour. He then got better, and for a few months was able to do a little light work. He could not, however, walk without the assistance of two sticks. After some time he became an in-patient of Exeter hospital for four weeks, and then an out-patient for one week more. He derived considerable benefit from the remedies applied at the institution, but the relief was only temporary; for after a few months he relapsed, and was again entirely incapable of

labour, and became so helpless that he was even unable to raise food to his mouth. The neighbouring farmers, taking compassion on him, raised a sum by subscription and bought him a donkey-cart, and for about six years he earned his subsistence by travelling about the country, when he was able, collecting rags and old metal. He was constantly obliged to make use of two sticks to assist him in walking. During the whole period of his illness he never received full wages. About Christmas, 1847, he happened to meet Mr. Capern in Newport Street, Tiverton. Mr. C., having heard his statement, invited him into the stable-yard of an adjoining house, and made the usual passes over the parts most affected, commencing at the back. Great and almost immediate benefit was experienced, and after two or three more operations he was completely cured. In two or three weeks he was in full work, and in receipt of the usual labourer's wages. In the early part of last summer he cut two acres of grass in one day. Occasionally, during changes of weather, he suffers slightly from rheumatic pains. Some weeks ago, having strained himself when at work, he came into Tiverton to see Mr. Capern, who by a few passes afforded him complete relief. With this exception, he has continued up to the present day quite well and strong.

Tiverton, October, 1849.

22. JOHN ROWDEN, agricultural labourer, aged 49, was a sufferer from severe rheumatic pain in the right hip for upwards of fourteen years. His complaint did not keep him from work, but in wet, damp, and cold

weather, and particularly during the prevalence of easterly winds, the pain was at times excruciating. On his first getting into bed at night it was usually very severe; but as the body acquired warmth it gradually became less and less, so that his nights were comparatively easy and his rest was not disturbed. During the whole period of his illness he was never entirely free from pain: for upwards of three years he was unable to stoop down, so as to unlace his boots; he could not have done it, he declares, if any body had offered him fifty pounds. He limped a good deal in his gait. He never had any medical advice; but had a variety of remedies recommended to him by different persons, but with no good result. While he was in this state, he happened one morning, as he was going to work, to meet Mr. Capern, to whom he was quite unknown, near the gate of Messrs. Heathcoat and Co.'s factory. He was then in a state of great suffering, and Mr. C., observing his lameness, invited him into the lodge, telling him he thought he might perhaps be able to do him some good. He accordingly accompanied Mr. C. into the lodge, not having the least idea what was going to be done to him as he had never heard of mesmerism or of Mr. C.'s mesmeric operations, which were then quite in their infancy. Almost immediately that the passes were made he experienced a strong sensation of heat in the limb and foot, as if, to follow his own description, something was making its way down the inside of the thigh and leg, which seemed to him as if they were "bumping." In two minutes, according to his own statement, all the pain was gone, he was able to stand with perfect ease upon the leg on the affected side and to use it freely; and went off to his work at such a pace as almost to distancc Mr. C., who was thrown into a considerable state of perspiration by his efforts to keep up with his patient. Since that time the pain has never returned with anything like its former violence. Occasionally during wet or cold weather, or when the wind is easterly, he feels it slightly; but his sufferings on such occasions are a mere nothing in comparison with those which he formerly endured. His lameness still remains with no material improvement.

23. WILLIAM WEBBER, agricultural labourer, in the employ of Mr. Cook, of Barton, was hurled down by a horse, about two years ago, as he was attending at a sale, and much bruised and hurt in the right arm and shoulder. He applied to a surgeon who gave him some oil to rub into the limb; as this afforded him no relief, he had recourse to another medical man; but with a similar and unsuccessful result. He suffered greatly. The limb was much discoloured, and there was an almost total loss of power. He was hardly able to move his arm, and declares that he could not have lifted anything from the table, far less have raised it to his lips, if the whole world had been offered to him. After remaining two or three weeks in this state without the least improvement, except that the arm had almost recovered its natural colour, he was advised by his master, Mr. Monday, of Greenham, to apply to Mr. Capern. He came into Tiverton on a Wednesday, and remained until the Saturday following, when he returned home.

The pain was then almost entirely gone, and he was able to raise food to his lips without difficulty or inconvenience. He came into town three times in the following week, at the end of which period he was completely cured and able to return to his work.

October 17th, 1850.

24. THOMAS WILLIAMS, of Bickleigh, suffered for four months from rheumatism. After the third operation on him by Mr. Capern he was completely cured and able to return to his labour, and he has had no return of it since.

25. ROBERT HILL, in the employ of Thomas Carew, Esq., 45 years of age. About two years and a quarter since he had severe rheumatic pains for from eight to ten weeks. He walked sometimes with one and sometimes with two sticks. He applied to a surgeon, and used the means recommended without any benefit. He afterwards applied to Mr. Capern, and got to his house with difficulty. He was quite disabled from work. Mr. C. made some passes on him, after which he was able to walk in the garden without his sticks; he could even have walked home without them. The change was so great that his neighbours were astonished to see him. He applied to Mr. Capern twice afterwards, and was operated on, and he has not lost a day's work since. Until he applied to Mr. Capern he was obliged to go up stairs to bed upon his hands and knees. He is now as free from pain as ever he was in his life.

26. George Candy, limeburner, Elmore, Tiverton, aged 55, was subject from his twentieth year to frequent attacks of rheumatism; suffering much pain, and often disabled from following his occupation. On one of those occasions he had been three weeks on crutches when he happened accidentally to meet with Mr. Capern near a public house about a quarter of a mile from his own house. He requested Mr. C. to try whether he could do him any good. Mr. C. consented, and went with him into the parlour of the public house and commenced the passes. He felt some immediate relief whilst this was being done; and, as he was proceeding homewards, he suddenly recovered the full use of his limbs, and was able to walk with ease and comfort to his own house, carrying his crutches in triumph over his shoulders. He contracted a cold in consequence of imprudent exposure; had a return of the pain in his ancles, and was entirely confined to his bed for five or six weeks, unable to lift a limb, owing to the great suffering caused by the least motion. He was under constant medical treatment, but experienced little or no relief. His bill for medicine and attendance amounted to five pounds fourteen shillings. At the end of the period named he again had recourse to Mr. Capern, and after several operations his health was entirely restored, and he has never had a return of the complaint since, with the exception of a slight pain in the knee that was immediately removed by a few passes by Mr. Capern. He is now quite well, and to all appearance a hale, healthy, and exceedingly active man. It is nearly three years

since the first cure was effected, and about four or five months since he was the second time relieved.

27. WILLIAM MIDDLE, of Cullompton, painter and glazier; had been afflicted with rheumatic gout for from ten to twelve years. He was frequently disabled from working at his trade. He first applied to Mr. Capern on Sunday, September 9th, 1849, being then unable to move his leg, except by taking hold of it and raising it with both his hands. Even with this precaution the movement caused pain. He rose from his chair with difficulty, and usually only after many ineffectual attempts to do so. His nights were almost sleepless, and he had very little appetite. He only left his bed, where he had been confined for eight weeks, the Thursday previous; and from the immense swelling of the knee, the general prostration of strength, and the intense pain which he suffered, he believed that he would be altogether disabled from work for the future. He could not walk without assistance over the threshold of his door. His only mode of getting up stairs was to rest one knee upon the step above him, and then drag up the affected leg with it. Standing for any time, or any exertion, caused great exhaustion and a copious sweating. For the last twelve months he had been unable to pull off his stockings without assistance, and for six months of that time to lift his leg on the bed. When he retired to rest, his stockings were always pulled off and his leg raised and laid on the bed for him by his wife or some other person. A little girl was sent with him to Tiverton, for the express purpose of performing those accustomed

services; but her aid was never required, as after the first mesmerisation he was able to manage without any difficulty by himself. During his illness he had had the benefit of the advice of five or six medical men, and tried a variety of remedies without effect. Contact passes with the flat of the hand were made over the left shoulder and arm for about seven minutes, and then in the same manner down the leg on the affected side. He soon felt an unusual glow of heat, and in about twelve minutes after the commencement of the treatment was relieved from all pain, and able to move his leg freely, and even to lift and place it with ease upon the table before him. On the same afternoon he walked more than a mile, without the least assistance of a stick, with no pain, and with more ease and freedom than he had experienced for many years. There was an immediate improvement in his sleep and appetite. On going out into the air, about twenty minutes after the first mesmerisation, he was suddenly seized with a violent shaking of the limbs and chattering of the teeth. This lasted about half an hour, and then went off spontaneously. He continued to be mesmerised twice every day during his stay in Tiverton, and with rapid and decided improvement. On the eighth day he returned home quite free from pain, with no stiffness of the limbs, and able to walk about all day without fatigue, or sweating, or any inconvenience whatever. His appetite was good, he slept long and soundly at night, and in fact there was nothing left of his former symptoms but the swelling of the knee, which was much reduced. It was his intention to resume his work on the following day.

August 13th.—He was engaged in his employ as painter, beautifying Cullompton Tower, and ascended a ladder fifty feet high.

28. Mrs. Mary Tapp, aged 60, was afflicted upwards of fifteen years with violent pains in the head, arms, hips, and thighs. During the whole of this period she was never entirely free from pain. She was often unable to obtain any rest at night, in consequence of her sufferings, which were at times so severe as to oblige her to leave her bed and endeavour to find relief in motion or change of position. She was rendered altogether incapable of any laborious exertion, and unable to take any active part in the management of her farm-yard. Sometimes for weeks together she suffered so much that she was unable to comb her hair or lace her stays without assistance. Happening to be accidentally at Mr. Capern's on some business when one of Mr. C.'s patients was being mesmerised, and seeing the great relief afforded by the passes, she was induced to ask him to try what he could do for her. She had very little expectation of receiving benefit from his exertions, since from her advanced age and the long duration of her sufferings she had been led to look upon her case as hopeless. The first attempt was followed by the almost entire cessation of pain in the limbs. She did not see Mr. C. again until after an interval of some weeks, when by the passes being made over the head the pains in that part were also entirely removed. Afterwards she was mesmerised three or four times, the passes being continued about ten or twelve minutes

each time. She now considers herself cured. She takes the active management of the farm-yard, performing the operation of milking her cows, which for many years she was totally unable to do. She works hard and suffers no inconvenience from the exertion. There is still a certain degree of stiffness in the fingers and elbow-joint on the side which was principally affected; but in general she is entirely free from pain, and although, when the weather is unfavourable, symptoms of her old complaint do now and then return, the attacks are so slight that they do not interfere with her work and she thinks little or nothing of them. It is now three years since the cure was effected.

January 17th, 1850.

29. Statement of Mr. Edwards, Prospect Place, Tiverton :—

"FRANCIS EDWARDS, son of Phoceon Edwards, was suffering for four years frequent attacks of rheumatism in the knee and leg, and at times prevented from walking without the assistance of a stick. He applied various remedies without producing any beneficial result, and looked forward to his entire incapacity for labour or exertion, the disease appearing to gain the ascendency, until nearly three years since, when I named it to Mr. Capern, who unhesitatingly offered to use his exertions to relieve my son, assuring me that he had confidence in his powers. At the first mesmerisation there was produced a general, comfortable heat, and an improvement. At the second, a considerable progress was made in the right direction: and after the third there was a total and an entire alleviation of pain, as well as an additional strength to that side of the body. This took place about three years since, and I have never heard him complain from that time. There had been a considerable swelling of the knee that subsided. Previously to the first operation he could not walk up and down the stairs without assistance."

Dec. 1st, 1849.

30. Samuel Doble, whitesmith, Gold Street, about twenty-four years since received a blow on the left leg from a heavy sledge hammer, wielded by one of his fellow-workmen. The small bone of the leg was broken, and inflammation of the part subsequently came on. A few months afterwards he was suddenly attacked by a severe pain in the same limb. He continued subject to similar attacks ten or twelve times a year. They always came on without warning, and sometimes when he was walking in the street or engaged in his usual occupation, so that he was obliged to be assisted home. On one occasion he was suddenly attacked whilst on a ladder, engaged in carrying up about twenty pounds of solder in a state of fusion, that he was obliged to throw down, whilst he himself had to be assisted to the ground by some of his fellow-workmen. The attacks sometimes lasted two or three weeks, and the pain was very severe. During their continuance he was disabled from attending to his work, and was generally confined to his house and frequently to his bed. He never had any medical advice, but tried a variety of remedies without improvement. A few years since he was engaged working at

his trade in a house not far from that in which Mr. Capern then resided; and Mr. C., finding him one morning in great pain and hardly able to move about, offered to operate upon him. He had been at work all the preceding night. Contact passes with the palm of the hand being made down over the seat of pain, he found immediate relief, accompanied with much warmth in the limb, and a pricking or tingling sensation in the soles of the feet. In less than five minutes the pain had entirely ceased. He had no return of it for nearly three years. About six weeks ago Mr. Capern accidentally met him in the street, and hearing that he was suffering from a slight return of his old pain, in consequence of an accidental cold, offered to make the passes over him; and in a few minutes entirely relieved him. The pain has not since then returned.

Dec. 24th. 1849.

31. John Williams, Backswood, Tiverton, had severe rheumatic pains in the back, shoulder, and legs, for five years and upwards; at times so bad that he could not walk across the room without the use of sticks; and he was totally unable to do any kind of labour. He applied various remedies, but without effect. At last he was advised to apply to Mr. Capern, which he did and he felt great relief from the first operation; and after a second the pains totally left him, and he has been free from them ever since.

32. James Summers.—"I live at Sampford Peverell, and was suffering continuous and acute pains in the hip-

joint and legs upwards of five weeks, insomuch that I was not able to walk across the house at times. On application to my medical attendant he stated that it probably originated from a chill, and believed it to be rheumatic affection. From him I took many doses of medicine, and was bled; but receiving no benefit I applied to Mr. Capern, who with pleasure instantly mesmerised the affected side. A comfortable heat was produced, and instantaneous relief, and I was astonished at the ease I experienced on returning to Sampford. A short time after I again stated to Mr. Capern that I had sensations of pain, although greatly alleviated. My friend again operated on me, which caused an entire cessation of pain. This last mesmerisation took place two years since, and I have been entirely and wholly free from that complaint, or any other, ever since, and can perform any kind of manual labour without inconvenience.

"JAMES SUMMERS.

"Oct. 28th, 1849."

33. GEORGE BEWY of Holcombe was, about six months since, seized with a violent attack of rheumatism. In consequence of his inability to labour he was obliged to leave his employer, Mr. Bowden of Allers. He was entirely cured by Mr. Capern after a few operations.

34. JOHN GILL, Cadeleigh, aged 53, was afflicted with rheumatism for many years. He walked with great difficulty to Tiverton to visit Mr. Capern, supported by two sticks. After a few passes he was able to walk back without them.

35. RICHARD STONE, of Uffculme, had been afflicted with rheumatism for three years, and had tried all kinds of medicines without any benefit. On his first application to Mr. Capern he felt immediate relief.

36. GEORGE LOWER, baker, Tiverton, in consequence of frequently leaving open the mouth of the oven, and amusing himself by fishing in the Exe whilst in a state of perspiration, took a chill, which deprived him of his sight. Severe rheumatism also settled in his legs. He suffered the most excruciating pain. A surgeon was applied to, under whose care he remained nine months; but there was no permanent improvement, only some temporary alleviation of his sufferings. Mr. Capern was sent for, and he felt great benefit at the first mesmerisation, and was perfectly restored in twelve or thirteen weeks.

37. SAMUEL HALL, agricultural labourer, in consequence of frequent exposure to the weather was a great sufferer from rheumatism. He was at times wholly incapable of labour, and when employed was never entirely free from pain. About two years and a half since he was induced to apply to Mr. Capern. For six months previous to that time his suffering had been particularly severe. Immediate relief was experienced from the passes, and he has remained free from pain ever since.

38. ELIZABETH BECK, Newport Street, aged 70 years, was suffering rheumatic pains continually for five

years, in the shoulders and arm, insomuch as at times to be incapable of attending to her domestic affairs or transacting any ordinary business. Her nights were generally restless, and the one previous to applying to Mr. Capern was sleepless. Immediately on the passes being made over the shoulder and arm she experienced an unusual degree of heat and relief from pain; and after three sittings all pain disappeared, and the consequence was undisturbed rest. This took place nearly three years since, and she has had no return of the complaint from that time.

Jan. 4th, 1850.

39. MRS. MITCHELL, wife of Mr. Mitchell, postmaster, Cullompton (statement received by Mr. Hopgood*), aged 56 years, a married woman with six children, states that at the age of 7 years she was attacked with rheumatism, which prevented any motion in the hip joint. She has never from that time until a fortnight since—a period of forty-nine years, been able to walk, except with the greatest difficulty and unremitting pain. She has constantly been under medical treatment, but without deriving any permanent benefit. Fourteen days since Mr. Capern began mesmerising her hip and leg. She described her sensations as being very peculiar, and causing a feeling of dread lest the hand of the operator should too suddenly be removed. She can now walk with scarcely any perceptible lameness, and without the slightest pain whatever, even when walking up and down stairs.

* Mr. Hopgood is a surgeon, retired from practice.

"The above statement of facts was related to me by the patient herself, who appears to be a person of truth and respectibility.

"JOSEPH HOPGOOD.

"Exe Villa,
August 29th, 1849."

40. Statement of ROBERT PARKER, agricultural labourer, Stoodleigh, aged 56 years.

"For the last twelve months I have been suffering from severe rheumatic pains down the right side and leg, which prevented my taking my daily labour for a considerable time. On the 30th of November I applied to Mr. Capern, of Tiverton, who afforded me great relief; and I have applied to him twice since, and now consider myself quite cured. On my first visit I walked to Tiverton with great difficulty with the assistance of two sticks; before my return home I found I could dispense with them, and have not bcen obliged to use them since. My earnings for the last four months have been only fifteen shillings."

41. ISAAC QUICK, aged 56 years, agricultural labourer, Cove, had suffered from severe rheumatic pain in the left arm for five or six days. He was unable to remain in bed for five minutes at a time, but spent the night either sitting up in a chair or lying in his clothes outside the bed. He had not slept for half an hour from his first attack to the time of his making application to Mr. Capern. After the first operation, the pain was

much mitigated. He was mesmerised in all five times, at intervals of some days, with continued improvement. After the fifth operation he considered himself cured. He ceased to attend and has had no return of pain since.

42. SARAH QUICK, wife of the above, aged 53 years, had suffered for several years from rheumatic pains in the hip and leg. She was always in pain; and in cold, wet, or damp weather her sufferings were very severe. She was mesmerised by Mr. Capern four times, after which the pain entirely left her.

Copy of a letter received from Mr. William Gunn, schoolmaster, of Oakford.

"Agreeably to the request contained in yours of the 26th ulto., I have called on the individuals therein named, Mrs. Wyburn, Mrs. Mogford, and Mr. Carpenter, of this parish, and have great satisfaction in forwarding to you their statements; and, if these are intended for publication, I could furnish you with more lengthy particulars. I am requested by the parties to express to you their gratitude for your exertions, which in each of their cases have proved successful; and they consider that they can never sufficiently repay you for your disinterested kindness, but offer up their prayers that you may have sufficient strength to carry out your benevolent intentions. I am convinced that you feel delighted at affording relief to suffering humanity, and I hope, from the prayers of the great number you have relieved, that Providence may continue to bless you with the extraordinary power which you possess, and which has been developed in the face of scepticism and doubt. Let me entreat you not to relinquish your exertions in consequence of the aspersions and insults to which you have been subjected. I have heard of them with deep concern and lament that after the sacrifices you have made for several years you should receive such insult; but, sir, remember that justice will eventually be done. Wishing you if possible an increase of power and strength.

"I am, Sir, yours, &c.,
"WILLIAM GUNN."

[Copy. Statement.]

43. "MRS. WYBURN, Oakford, was afflicted with dreadful pains in her feet and legs. The sinews were drawn up for six months before applying to Mr. Capern to such a degree that she could take no rest all night, and was in the most excruciating pains imaginable. After the first time the passes were made she could sleep soundly, and after the fourth time the pains were entirely gone: with gratitude to Mr. Capern,

"MARY WYBURN."

(Witness) William Gunn.

44. MR. CARPENTER says "that he was troubled with rheumatic pains for eight months previous to applying to Mr. Capern. That he could take no rest by night and scarcely crawl about by day; that after the first time his rest returned, and at the sixth time,

although 73 years of age, the pain was nearly eradicated.

"The mark of × WILLIAM CARPENTER."

(Witness) William Gunn.

45. MRS. MOGFORD says "that she was afflicted for some time with acute pains in her legs; that after the passes were made a few times the pains were completely removed, and she has not felt them since.

"MARY MOGFORD."

(Witness) William Gunn.

46. Statement from Samuel Viney, Tiverton.

"This is to certify that I, Samuel Viney, aged 56 years, was attacked with a violent pain in my right shoulder, in the year 1847, which continued nearly four weeks. I applied to Mr. Thomas Capern, in Tiverton; who by his stroking my shoulder once completely cured me, and I have not felt the least symptom of it since.

"SAMUEL VINEY."

47. JOHN NORRISH, shoemaker, Hammett's Lane, Tiverton, aged 17 years, states "that whilst amusing myself with other youths I was thrown into the river Lowman, from which I took a chill, which brought on severe rheumatism and prevented me from labour. I was attended by surgeons here who did not afford me any relief. I obtained a recommendation to the Exeter hospital, but such was the nature and severity of the complaint that they neither did nor attempted to relieve me. They gave me no medicine nor put me into baths.

After remaining one month, I came out pronounced as incurable. I applied to Mr. Capern on a Friday: when he first made the passes I felt relief, and by their being repeated the Sunday week following the pains left me, and I am now quite recovered. There was a consultation of seven surgeons at Exeter."

48. CHARLES SYDENHAM, Hammett's Lane, Tiverton, states,—"I suffered from rheumatic pain several months, but, after the passes had been made a few times, I quite recovered, and have had no return of them from that time.

49. Mrs. QUICK, wife of John Quick, Townsend, states,—"I suffered violent pain in my head and face for twelve months. I felt relief after the passes were first made, and, after three or four times repeating, I was quite recovered."

50. RICHARD, son of the above, suffered from rheumatism in the feet, and was subject to fits for three or four months. He could scarcely walk. From repeated application of the passes, in less than a month he was quite restored.

51. THOMAS PRESCOTT, Bampton, suffered rheumatic pains for several years. He applied to a surgeon, but received no benefit. He suffered greatly during the month previous to applying to Mr. Capern. He felt better after the first sitting, and after the fourth he was completely cured.

52. ELIZABETH WOTTON, Cheriton Fitzpaine, had a sudden attack of rheumatism in the knee at night, in consequence of which she was obliged to leave her service. She applied to a medical man, but received no relief. She applied to Mr. Capern, and in five minutes she experienced more relief than she had for the six preceding weeks. After one more sitting she left Tiverton for the purpose of taking her situation again.

53. CAROLINE VESEY, aged 21 years, farm servant to Mr. Chubb, parish of Halberton, was working in a field, hay-making, nearly two years ago, and, being very warm, sat down to milk the cows; when she took a chill which gave her severe rheumatism in the hips, back, and loins. She had medical advice frequently, but derived no permanent relief. She suffered a great deal of pain, and was obliged to leave her situation. Several times her mother wished her to go to the Exeter Hospital. Her mistress recommended her to go to Mr. Capern, as he had cured a great many and might do her good. She followed her advice, and was mesmerised by Mr. C. on Tuesday se'night, and experienced immediate relief from the pain: but the lameness still remained, and she went to Mr. Capern on the following Friday, and was mesmerised twice; when she was able to walk home without any pain or inconvenience. This Tuesday she returned to thank Mr. C. and gave him this statement.

April 9th, 1850.

54. Mr. RICHARD PONSFORD, yeoman, aged 67

years, parish of Moreborth, has been suffering from rheumatism and rheumatic gout for more than twenty years. The attacks were generally most severe during the winter, confining him to his room, and frequently to his bed. He was often under medical treatment, but never received any permanent relief. Being in Tiverton one market day, two months ago, he by accident saw Mr. Capern cure a poor man of rheumatism by mesmerism, which made so great an impression on him that he immediately intreated Mr. Capern to operate upon him in a similar manner. Mr. C. kindly consenting, a few mesmeric passes were made over his leg and thigh, from which he experienced immediate relief. At this date he has been operated upon five times, for about seven minutes each time, and he now sleeps well at night, and has no inconvenience in walking, although the limb is smaller than the other and slightly contracted.

Tiverton, April 2nd, 1850.

55. William King, aged 16 years, farm servant to Mr. John Summers, parish of Sampford Peverell, fell over a hurdle about four months ago and hurt his left leg severely. Next day he got wet, and this brought on rheumatism in the injured part. He applied to the parish doctor, who ordered it to be bathed twice a day and gave him some medicine; but he received no great benefit and was confined to his bed for nine weeks. The boy's master recommended the mother frequently to take him to Mr. Capern, who had cured him, Mr. Summers, and he was sure Mr. C. could do her son

good. She did so on Friday the 6th inst., and drove him in a little donkey-cart to Mr. Capern's door; he being unable to walk and suffering great pain. He was mesmerised for about five minutes; and experienced great relief from the operation. His mother was induced to leave him until Tuesday, and he was operated upon twice each day during the interval, and is now free from pain and able to return to his work.

Tiverton, April 9th, 1850.

56. Richard Clarke, aged 14 years, servant to Mr. John Tucker, Washfield, was suddenly seized about a month ago with a very severe rheumatic pain in the right knee, that confined him to his bed for more than a week, and he could neither move nor turn without suffering the most excruciating agony. While in this state, he was attended by the parish doctor and took by his directions medicine every four hours. This afforded him partial relief, and he was in a few days able to leave his bed: but his leg had become contracted and he could not walk without great pain and lameness, and his father thought he would be a cripple for life. On Sunday, the 27th January, he was taken into Tiverton, for the purpose of seeing Mr. Capern; and, meeting that gentleman accidentally in the street, was taken by him to his house, when the usual mesmeric passes were made on his leg and knee, and in less than ten minutes he was relieved from pain. He then accompauied Mr. Capern a short distance, to the residence of a gentleman to whom Mr. C. wished to shew him. He had no difficulty in walking, though still lame from the stiffness of

the leg. He was again operated upon. Great warmth was felt in the limb, especially about the knee; and he walked about the room with still less lameness than before. On the 31st he again returned to Tiverton. The lameness was gone, and he declared his intention of resuming his work next day.

57. MARY SNOW, aged 60, parish of Sampford Peverell, had suffered for two years from severe pains in, and enlargement of, the knee-joint. She tried many remedies, but without any beneficial effects. Her husband, having heard that Mr. Capern of Tiverton had cured a great many persons of various complaints, pressed her repeatedly to apply to that gentleman, but she was fearful of so doing as she had heard a great many very extraordinary reports about "mesmerism." But, one day accidentally meeting Mr. Capern, he invited her into the house of a female friend whom he had cured a few days before of tic douloureux. He then passed his hand about half a dozen times over her knee, and she felt the pain leave the knee and gradually descend, following his hands, and passing out at the toe. The swelling shortly after disappeared, and she has had no return of it since. Before going into the house with Mr. Capern her heart almost failed her; so much was she afraid of "mesmerism."

58. ROBERT CHANNING, of Stoodleigh, yeoman, was subject to severe attacks of rheumatism for above ten years; and for the four years previous to being operated upon by Mr. Capern his sufferings were very great

—at times almost unbearable, so as to incapacitate him from attending to his business on the farm. He had almost invariably restless nights. The first time he was operated upon he felt an improvement; and, after three sittings, he was entirely free from pain. He has continued so ever since, except at change of weather, when he occasionally suffers a slight inconvenience. A few passes from Mr. Capern instantly restore him to ease. He was operated upon nearly three years since.

January, 1850.

59. WILLIAM POPE, yeoman, of Tiverton, aged 50 years, was attacked about four months ago with a severe pain in his right arm, that afterwards extended to the neck and shoulder of the same side. He suffered most at night when he became warm in bed, and was often unable to turn without great difficulty and severe pain. On Tuesday the 5th February he applied to Mr. Capern, who by mesmerising his arm for a few minutes relieved him from all pain, and he was able to move and use it with more freedom than he had done since the attack. Before the operation the pulse was seventy-two, but after it only sixty-seven.

60. WILLIAM PATTISON, Haddon Hill, Somerset, aged 25 years, was for four years a great sufferer from rheumatic pains principally in the legs. For the first year and a half of this time he was entirely incapacitated from work; and during the whole time of his illness he was unable to put on his clothes without assistance. He found no relief from medicine, although he had

recourse to a variety of remedies. During the last two years and a half he was able to go about with a little more ease, and occasionally to do some light work; but he could not walk two miles without suffering great pain afterwards in the feet and legs, nor could he make any exertion with the limb without suffering from it. By the first mesmerisation he was very much benefited. During the next five weeks he did almost as much work as in the whole previous twelvemonth. He was able also to walk many miles without pain or suffering any inconvenience from the exertion. His general health was also greatly improved. A few passes were made over him three times afterwards, at intervals of some weeks, and he is now completely cured.

61. Mrs. Pattison, mother of the above, was also a great sufferer from rheumatism for about seven years: during which time she was often laid up by it. By the first operation she was very much benefited. The pain was entirely removed and she was able to walk better than she had done for a twelvemonth before. There was no return of the pain until about four weeks afterwards, when she accidentally caught a cold, in consequence of which she felt a slight return of stiffness in the leg. She again applied to Mr. C. and was mesmerised for about ten minutes. The relief afforded was immediate. The pain was entirely removed, and she walked with much more ease and freedom. She has been mesmerised but once since and is now quite well.

62. John Hayman, aged 18 years, parish of Tiver-

ton, was hay-making in the month of June last year, when he was suddenly seized with a severe rheumatic pain in the ankle of the right foot, and had great difficulty in reaching his own house. From that time until eight weeks passed he was quite unable to leave his bed. He was attended by a surgeon, and took powders sometimes every hour, and sometimes two or three times a day, but without any beneficial effect. About the end of the seventh week, a Mrs. Hawkins visited him and advised him to send for Mr. Capern, who, she informed him, had cured a great many cases of rheumatism. He therefore begged his mother to do so; but she not having any faith in mesmerism would not at first, and it was only at his repeated solicitation, and after a delay of several days, that she consented to do so. Mr. C. on visiting him made some passes on the part affected: this relieved him from all pain, and he had no return for several days. At the end of that time, however, the pain returned, but not so severely. He then sent a second time for Mr. C., who continued to attend him for about a week: at the end of which time he was completely cured. He has never had a return of the pain since.

63. Statement received from Mr. John Hatswell, St. Andrew's Street, Tiverton.

"About two years since I was attacked with inflammation in the chest, and was obliged to employ a medical man: it turned to rheumatic gout. I received no relief until I applied to Mr. Capern, and after a few passes I found the greatest benefit. In the course of the year I was again attacked with rheumatism, and made a similar application with the same success. About a month since I fell from a horse and dislocated my shoulder. I again applied to Mr. C and found immediate relief.

"JOHN HATSWELL,
"St. Andrew's Street.

"Tiverton, 20th Dec., 1849."

64. SAMUEL PAVORD, aged 4 years, suffered from pain and lameness in the right knee. His parents were advised to take him to Mr. Capern to be mesmerised. They did so and he was cured in six or seven minutes. He has remained well ever since.

65. SARAH KINGDON, aged 53 years, parish of Rackenford, has suffered for about a twelvemonth from severe pain and swelling in the right ankle and foot, and was often confined to her bed for seven or eight weeks at a time. She lost the use of her ankle, her foot hanging quite useless. She has been under surgical treatment but without benefit. Her husband, hearing of the cures performed by Mr. Capern, brought her into Tiverton to him, and she is now under mesmeric treatment. The pain is quite gone and she is gradually recovering the use of her foot. She was also suffering from deafness; but since she has been under his care her hearing is also improved.

66. PHILIP HODGE, parish of Netherexe, aged 75, agricultural labourer, states that he has been suffering at intervals from severe attacks of rheumatic gout for

the last twenty years. He has been frequently confined to his bed for four or five consecutive weeks; and for the greater part of this period he has not been able to walk without the assistance of a stick; and such was his weakness that after being confined to his bed he was compelled to walk with crutches. Since Christmas last he has been incapable of performing one day's labour and has suffered considerably; in fact, at times he could not stand erect in consequence of the pains in the back. Mr. Capern having benefited his wife and son-in-law, Samuel Brittan, he was induced to apply to Mr. C., and came to Tiverton for the purpose of being operated upon. Mr. C. commenced making the passes down the back and side on Wednesday, the 22nd May. There was a comfortable glow of heat experienced, and every successive operation has produced similar results and a gradual improvement; and on this day (April 29th) he is about to return home. He has now more ease and comfort than he has had for a long time, and is confident that if necessary he could walk to his home, a distance of nine miles, without the assistance of a stick. His general health also is improved.

67. Mary Welsh, Cullompton, July 15th, 1849. Statement. "It is now about two years since I applied to you for the dropsy and rheumatic affection; as for the dropsy, I am happy to say I am quite recovered through the means of you and no other person; as for the rheumatism which I have been suffering in all my lifetime, I am considerably better and still amending. After trying various means to no effect, I applied to you,

and I am willing to testify to any person. My age is about 54 years.

"I am, Sir,

"MARY WELSH.

"To Mr. T. Capern."

68. Statement of JOHN LETHBRIDGE, labourer, Westexe.—"Whilst at work in a hay-field, occupied by Mr. Ford, in the summer of 1847, I felt a sudden attack of inflammation of the knee. The swelling was so rapid that my friends were compelled to cut my clothes from me. I was confined to my bed and under the surgeon's care for six weeks. From thence I was removed to the Exeter Hospital, where I was a patient nine weeks. There was also a contraction of the muscles of the knee. An issue was inserted near the knee; and thirty peas were placed daily in it for the purpose of opening a wound. This caused me great pain. At the time of my leaving, a consultation of surgeons was held and the case pronounced hopeless and incurable, and they stated that I should be crippled for life. I was compelled to walk with two sticks. I met with Mr. Capern in Westexe, and he, observing the pain and difficulty I had in walking, offered to make a few passes over me, which he did, and in five minutes I was enabled to walk without the assistance of any stick. Within a few weeks the pains left me; but the stiffness was not removed for ten or twelve weeks; after which time I was enabled to resume my daily labour, and am now as well as ever I was in my life."

69. The following testimonial was received from Mr. John Berry, dated, Torquay, July 1st, 1850;—

"Dear Sir,—I was afflicted with rheumatism over the whole of my frame, and whilst residing near Bath made applications to several medical gentlemen there, whose efforts proved unsuccessful. I then obtained an order and was admitted as a patient into the General Bath Hospital, where I received a little benefit. I was then advised to apply to you, which I very willingly did, and after a few passes at the first sitting I received more relief than I had experienced for five months previous from all the surgeons at Bath, or the Bath waters; in fact I was enabled to place my hand on my head which I had not done since the attack. From that time I have had no relapse, and at present am quite capable of attending to my duties. I feel happy through divine providence in sending you this testimonial of your charitable exertions towards the afflicted, that you might make use of it in any way you may think proper.

"I am, Sir, your obedient servant,

"John Berry."

70. John Wolland, labourer of Broad Lane, Tiverton in the employ of the Rev. John Spurway, states, That five years since, he had very severe pains in the right knee; he applied to a surgeon, who gave an opinion that the muscles of the knee were sprained, and applied three blisters to the parts affected. The application afforded a slight relief. He was then advised by his friends to go to the Exeter Hospital. He, however, saw Mr. Capern, who offered to operate on him, and

did; and after ten or twelve sittings he was relieved from pain, and continues so, except a slight inconvenience on the change of weather.

71. James Coles:—

The following statement is from James Coles, agricultural labourer, of Bampton Down:—"I was afflicted with rheumatic pains over the whole of my body for sixteen years, during which time the attacks were so severe that I was occasionally confined to my bed for weeks together (five at one time), and so helpless that I was incapable of dressing or undressing myself. About a month since I was advised to apply to Mr. Capern, of Tiverton, and I did on the 23rd of June last: and after a few passes being made over the arms and legs I felt warmth and ease, and in five minutes was released from pain. Since that time I have made two other applications to Mr. C. with the same success; and at the present time, through his kind perseverance, am enabled to resume my labour without the least pain, and consider myself quite well.

"Dated, 23rd July, 1850."

72. William Russell, Leat Street, Tiverton, aged 54 years, carpenter, whilst engaged at Honiton experienced at night violent pains in the leg and ankle, similar to cramp. He was unable to rest, and was compelled to walk about the room. Though still suffering considerable pain, he again retired to bed, and dressed himself in the morning with difficulty. On descending the stairs the attack became more violent, and, but for

the strength of the balusters he would have fallen down, being incapable of making any exertion of the instep, which was quite powerless: the foot dropping down as if the tendons had been severed. From Honiton he was brought to Tiverton in a gig, and was apprehensive that he would never be able to walk or work again. He remained in this melancholy condition with full health and vigour for thirteen weeks, until one morning Mr. Searles, builder, for whom he had frequently laboured, called at his house for the purpose of employing him, being in want of hands. Russell says—"I stated my inability to labour. A few minutes afterwards Mr. Capern called and said that he came at the request of Mr. Searles to operate on me; which he did, and within eight minutes I was relieved from pain and was able to put on my boots, which I had not attempted to do for the thirteen previous weeks. I immediately went to my labour. This took place nearly three years ago, and I have been invariably free from pain ever since."

73. ANN ESCOTT, Stoodleigh, aged 16 years, states that she had a sudden attack of severe pain in the arm, which for several weeks was completely paralyzed. She applied to a surgeon and a physician, but received no benefit: at length she was induced to apply to Mr. Capern, and after about twelve sittings she was completely cured.

74. SARAH POOK, Leat Street, Tiverton, was afflicted with severe rheumatic fever for three weeks. She suf-

fered extreme pain and could move neither hand, foot, nor neck; her right hand lay upon her breast, and she was incapable of moving a finger of it. She had medical advice, but without any improvement. Her mother, on being informed of her state, came in from the country to nurse her, and almost the first words she heard from her daughter were, "oh, mother, pray do send for Mr. Capern." Mr. C. obeyed the summons and went to see her. After the first operation the pain was much relieved, and she was able to move her fingers. She was mesmerised about fifteen or sixteen times more, and in five or six weeks a complete cure was effected.

75. "I, THOMAS ISAACS, late of Butterleigh, yeoman, aged 60 years, certify that four years since I was confined to my bed for thirteen weeks by typhus fever. By the great ravages made by it in my constitution, and by the weakness of my side, I was incapable of much exertion and had not sufficient strength to walk above half a mile at any time, and walking for even that distance produced increased debility; in fact, I considered I should be powerless during the remainder of my days. I was requested by several of my friends to apply to Mr. Capern for the purpose of being mesmerised; and after attending at his house a few times I had an increase of strength and less pain; and within a few weeks I was much better than I ever expected to be, and my nights which had been previously sleepless by reason of the pains in the legs and thighs were now painless and comfortable. This took place two years since, and the only thing I complain of now is a stiffness in the joints and

thighs that is immediately removed by a few passes over the affected joints."

76. Elizabeth Pope, Wellbrooke, aged 54 years, states,—"About twenty-seven years since I had a severe attack of fever, from which I lost the use of my limbs. I was troubled much with rheumatism and palpitation of the heart, extreme noise in the head, and deafness in one ear. I have been under various surgeons, but they did me no good; and I was in the Bristol hospital, from whence I was discharged as incurable. Until I applied to Mr. Capern I was not able to walk after my first attack without the aid of crutches, and then only on tip-toe. After a few applications to him I lost the deafness, and then I gradually got better, and am now able to walk about and do all my washing and domestic affairs; and, although living a considerable distance from the church, I have been able to walk there twice a day."

77. Elizabeth Goss, widow, Hammett's Lane, aged 64 years, was attacked nearly a month since with great pain underneath the arm; it then spread over the whole arm, and rendered her incapable of labour or even of any motion. From the shoulder a deadness pervaded, particularly the lower part of the arm and hand. She applied to a surgeon who gave her oils to rub in, but they afforded no relief. She was compelled to wear a glove when exposed to the open air, and to fold her arm in a shawl whilst in the house. She was induced

to apply to Mr. Capern in consequence of his having been instrumental in affording relief to her brother, John Binton, a few days after he had broken his leg. On the 30th of March last she had the passes made over her and felt relief; after two more sittings she was completely cured.

"Oakford, Sept. 6th, 1850.

78. "Dear Sir,—Agreeable to your request I have sent you the statement of Fanny Haskins as below.

"I remain,
"Yours respectfully,
"W. GUNN."

"Oakford, Sept. 6th, 1850.

"Sir, with gratitude to you for the great benefit you bestowed on me in restoring me to perfect health after nine months affliction in the most excruciating rheumatic pains; and after trying various medicines which was all to no purpose, I was persuaded to apply to you which resulted, I am happy to say, in a perfect cure, and that too with four visits only.

"I am, Sir,
"Yours gratefully,
"FANNY HASKINS.

"To Mr. Capern, Tiverton."

"Cullompton, Aug. 14th, 1850.

"Dear Sir,—I beg to send you the following statement, and sincerely thanking you for your kindness and attention to me and for the benefit I have received from you,

"I remain, dear Sir,

"Yours truly obliged,

"RICHARD TAPSCOTT.

"To Mr. Thomas Capern, Tiverton."

[Statement.]

79. "On the 12th August, 1842, Richard Tapscott, of Cullompton, in the county of Devon, writer, then 38 years old, met with an accident by which his hip bone was dislocated and his thigh fractured. He has since that time been a great sufferer from rheumatism, extending at times from the hip bone to the ankle. About two months ago he was fortunately in the company of Mr. Thomas Capern in Tiverton, and on rising from the place where he had been sitting, he complained very much of rheumatism, on which Mr. Capern asked him how it was occasioned, and, on being informed, said he could give him some relief. Mr. Capern then passed his hand outside the trousers, over the place affected, and, continuing the same for about the space of five minutes, the pain entirely ceased and has not since in the slightest degree returned.

"About three weeks ago he was again injured by a severe pressure in the back that caused a very violent pain or lumbago, so that he could scarcely walk for three or four days. He again fortunately met with Mr. Capern in Fore Street, Tiverton, who observed how badly he was walking, and, on being informed how it was occasioned, went with him to the Phœnix Inn, and, after passing his hand over the part affected for about three minutes, the pain entirely ceased and has not since returned. He is now as free from rheumatism as he was before his accident, and he sends this statement to Mr. Capern in order that by his publication of the same, others similarly afflicted may seek and obtain similar relief. Nothing whatever was done by Mr. Capern but slightly passing his hand over the part affected; and the sensation at the time was as if an hot iron had been passed over the part affected.

"RICHARD TAPSCOTT.

"Cullompton, Aug. 14th, 1850.

"To Mr. Thomas Capern,
"Tiverton, Devon."

80. ANN EASTERBROOK (wife of William Easterbrook, Cullompton, Devon, labourer), 55 years old.

"I have been severely afflicted with rheumatism for many years past, and have been attended by various doctors, but could get no relief from any of them. Upwards of a year and a half ago I heard of the cures of Mr. Capern of Tiverton. Previously to this I had been confined to my bed for nearly nine months with the rheumatism. I was taken over to Tiverton in a donkey cart to Mr. Capern's house. I was lifted out of the cart, and all but carried into Mr. Capern's house, being entirely unable to walk without assistance. After Mr. Capern had made passes with his hand over the part affected for about five minutes, he asked me if I could rise up. I did so, and put on my bonnet and walked without assistance, and without even using a stick, from

Mr. Capern's house down to Back Lane near the factory—a distance of more than a quarter of a mile. I felt entirely free from pain. This was about 11 o'clock in the forenoon. About 3 o'clock in the afternoon of the same day Mr. Capern came down to me in Back Lane, and made a second application of the passes for a few minutes. I then went to the public house where my donkey cart had been sent—a distance farther than from Back Lane to Mr. Capern's house. I walked there without a stick and without any other assistance. I can now go out to my daily labour and am entirely free from rheumatism.

"The mark + of ANNE EASTERBROOK.

"Witness to the mark of the said Anne Easterbrook, } RICHARD TAPSCOTT."

81. RICHARD DREWE, Sandford, near Crediton, in the employ of Mr. Thos. Lee, has suffered from sciatica for twelve months. Last half year his sufferings have been very great. He has suffered fearfully; could not walk without a stick, and with difficulty then. First operation by Mr. Capern on Monday, September 9th, 1850. Previous to first application could not sleep. After application free from pain and slept well. Thursday following could walk without a stick better than with two sticks before. Returned to his employ on the Saturday.

82. ANN TUCKER, Thoverton, but now residing at Tiverton, 57 years of age. "Have not been able to walk without a stick for about three years and a half,

and more particularly for the last six months, until about four months ago, when I applied to Mr. Capern. I have applied occasionally since, and can now walk without a stick and am completely cured of the rheumatics. I have a violent pain in my head and inside. After a few passes I feel great relief."

83. Statement of rheumatic gout by Dr. Richard Harrison Black ;—

"In company with Mr. Capern I visited Mrs. Sarah Webber, about 69 years of age, who, during the last seven years, had been unable to walk or even stand upright without great pain and difficulty. It was Mr. C.'s first visit. She stated that her principal pain was at the hip-joint. After a few passes she exclaimed, 'Oh, I am in such pain here (along the thigh) ; oh, it is so hot and in pain that is unbearable.' A short time after, the passes having been continued, she uttered a shout of joy, 'Blessed be God! all the pain is gone, and I feel I can stand up.' This she did, and for about a minute remained standing, looking intently on Mr. C., and then turning her eyes upwards as if in gratitude to heaven. With one hand only on the wall she walked along two sides of the room. Her neighbour, Mrs. Martin cried out, "God be praised! I have known Mrs. Webber for a long period, and never during that time knew her walk a step.' On the third day Mrs. W. said she could now rise without difficulty, which had not been the case for seven years. On the fourth she told me she had been continually walking about a little quite free from pain; and, every moment she moved, felt what a blessing had been granted her: can turn with ease in her bed, as well as ever in her life, which had not been the case for the last seven years. On the seventh day, Mrs. Martin saluted me with the exclamation, 'Mrs. Webber is quite well—that is, from the complaint for which application was made to Mr. C.;' and Mrs. W. in the most joyous tone said, 'Oh, what a delight to be out of pain: I never feel pain now, and can sleep as sound as any one.' Her visage on the first day was expressive of great anguish; on the seventh happiness was vividly depicted.

"October 24th. On calling to-day I found her at dinner. She exclaimed, 'Oh, Sir, I can now eat my meals right away without stopping, as I was obliged to do, and I can sleep right well at night; I was downright astonished to be awoke out of a right good sleep this morning by persons getting up. Before I saw Mr. Capern I heard almost every movement from night till morning.'

"October 28th. This morning I saw her, when she exclaimed, 'Oh, I feel stronger now, although I am near 69. I every day pray for Mr. Capern and the good persons that thought of this way of easing the pains of us poor people.'

"N.B. Very cold wind and wet had prevailed for the last two or three days which the prophets of ill declared would assuredly bring back all her pains.

"November 1st. Notwithstanding the evil predictions and the kind of weather which 'sorely,' as she said, 'tried her formerly,' this day in answer to the enquiry, 'How are you going on?' her reply was, 'I am quite happy and comfortable, and can enjoy everything, thank the Lord!'

"November 3rd. To-day Mrs. W. said, 'she was happy as any queen could be, for now she could do everything herself.' Mrs. Martin here observed, 'Ah, the value of the good Mrs. W. has received no one can tell; about three weeks ago it was quite dreadful to see the sufferings of the poor creature. This shews what a mighty good the Lord can accomplish through his instrument Mr. C. What a pity he is going away.

"RICHARD HARRISON BLACK."

84. ABRAHAM CANN, near Coleford, Devon, states that for many years he has had attacks of rheumatic gout, and for the last two years the disease has been so severe that at times he could not attend to his accustomed employ. His nights were restless and he had calculated that ere long he should be compelled to relinquish work. He could not walk without the assistance of a stick or sticks. Failing in obtaining relief from various remedies, he was induced, in consequence of knowing several persons whom Mr. Capern of Tiverton had cured, to visit that town. At the time of his arriving there, his pains were very great. He took up his abode at the Swan on a Monday, when Mr. Capern commenced his operations, and visited him twice daily until the Saturday following, when the disease was entirely cured. A sensation of heat was produced the second day, and each successive time the power was applied it was with increased benefit.

85. Mrs. Pitt, wife of Mr. Pitt, an officer in the Milbank Penitentiary, was suffering for several months from severe rheumatism in the lower extremities, insomuch that she was prevented from attending to her domestic affairs. She applied to a surgeon who used various remedies without producing any benefit. She was at length recommended to try her native air as he could suggest nothing more. She consequently left for Tiverton, and, after remaining with her friends some time and experiencing no benefit from the change, was induced to apply to Mr. Capern, who commenced the manipulations, and after the first day considerable warmth was effected, and every day produced good effects. A decided cure was the result within five weeks and she is now able to attend to hęr domestic concerns free from pain.

86. Mr. John Williams, Montserrat, about four years ago suffered a severe attack of lumbago. After the application of a remedy recommended to him by a friend he recovered, but two years afterwards he was again attacked by the same complaint. His sufferings were very great; walking or rising from the chair, or any movement whatever, caused him intense pain. He felt easy when completely at rest. On the third day after the commencement of the attack, feeling himself getting worse, he determined to go at once to the chemist who had made up the prescription which had relieved him previously, and have the same remedy prepared again. He told his wife before he set out that he was sure, if he did not go that day, he should not be able to go at

all. He was walking with great difficulty and in much pain, supported by two sticks, when he met Mr. Capern, whom he had known for some years. With some difficulty Mr. C. persuaded his friend to accompany him into a neighbouring house. Having ascertained the seat of pain, Mr. C. commenced making the usual passes with one hand; at the same time continuing the conversation, and Mr. Williams not having the least idea that he was being operated upon. Although Mr. Williams had heard of and often laughed at Mr. Capern's mesmeric operations, he had never been a witness of them, and was altogether ignorant of the mode of performing them. After sitting about ten minutes in this way, Mr. C. asked him to hand him a cup then on a table before them. Mr. Williams began to move his arm as usual very steadily and carefully, but, to his surprize, he felt no pain; much more was he astonished, when, on rising from his chair, he found that the pain had entirely left him; and that, to use his own expression, he was as well as ever he was in his life. "Why, Mr. Capern," he exclaimed, "I have no pain at all; what have you been doing to me?" He then learnt that he had been mesmerically operated upon. Instead of going to the chemist he returned home, when his wife was totally astonished to see him enter, walking as briskly and as well as ever. For some time she would not believe that he had had anything at all the matter with him, so sceptical was she upon the subject of mesmerism. The pain has never returned since. It should be mentioned that the mesmeric process caused Mr. Williams to fall into a violent perspiration.

July, 1850.

87. JAMES DAVEY, lime burner, Bampton, firstly had inflammation of the eyes. On its disappearance, about eight months since, he had severe pains in the back, that incapacitated him from labour for the whole time with the exception of one month. He applied to a surgeon; but, having received no benefit, he applied to two physicians in Exeter. One of them gave him a prescription from which he derived some benefit. However, he was induced to apply to Mr. Capern who made a few passes over the back and he felt more ease afterwards than during the previous eight months. He is now quite well.

SECTION II.

TIC DOULOUREUX OR NEURALGIA.

1. Copy of a letter received from Mr. Crocket of Collipriest.

"Tiverton, 24th July, 1850.

"Sir,—About two years ago I was suffering the most violent pains from tic douloureux, when I applied to you, and you were so kind as to make some mesmeric passes over my head that entirely removed the pain, and since that time I have not had a return of that complaint.

"I am, Sir, Yours obediently,

"JOHN CROCKER.

"To Mr. Capern."

2. SAMUEL BRITTON, agricultural labourer, Bampton Street, Tiverton, aged 50, about six years since, when descending a well seventy feet deep, was precipitated more than sixty feet to the bottom, in consequence of the handle of the windlass slipping through the hands of the person holding it. His left leg was broken into three pieces, and he was otherwise much bruised and hurt. He was obliged to submit to amputation of the limb. For three years he was able to do but little work, and he no sooner returned to full employment than he

had frequent attacks of excruciating pain in the stump. He was able to obtain but little rest; and was often obliged to leave his bed and walk about the room on crutches the whole night in consequence of his agonies. About two years ago, Mr. Capern happening to see him walking past his garden gate, and observing that it was with difficulty and apparently from pain, enquired what was the matter with him. After hearing the statement Mr. C. invited him into his house. This was in the afternoon. The man had gone to his work in the morning but had been compelled to leave it in consequence of his sufferings, and was then on his way home. He had never heard either of mesmerism or of Mr. Capern's cures. The usual passes were made over the limb, and in a few minutes the pain flew from the stump to the right shoulder, and then departed altogether, and never returned from that time. The patient has, however, been subject to occasional formation of abscesses in the stump that confined him to his house for weeks together and caused considerable pain. He never mentioned this to Mr. Capern until lately. A few passes being made down the stump on January 6th, 1850, a strong sensation of warmth was felt, which gradually descended till it appeared to the patient to reach the calf of the leg, and thence to go down to the extremities of the toes. He felt precisely the same sensations on the left side, when the passes were made over the stump, as he experienced in the right limb when the passes were made over the thigh on that side. A piece of rock crystal being drawn lengthways over the hand without contact, a prickling or tingling sensation was felt (see

Case of John Croote), and shortly afterwards severe pain and cramp in the elbow and shoulder joints. These sensations ceased after a few reverse passes up the arms by Mr. C.

Case in Paris.

3. Mr. George Wood, residing near Byron's Tavern, Rue Favert, on the Boulevards des Italiennes, states that on the 20th July he was thrown from his horse and severely injured his thumb; the whole arm was affected by this, more particularly the shoulder. He applied many remedies, and receiving no benefit was induced to apply to a surgeon, who ordered an application of some salve. He was apprehensive from the continued pain that he would have a locked jaw, more particularly on the night of the 23rd August. On the following day, being at a tavern, an English gentleman, observing that he was in pain and his thumb encased in leather, voluntarily offered to benefit him if he would allow it, and commenced operating by placing his hand on the shoulder and carrying it down the arm and hand. A degree of heat was perceptible, and the pains in the shoulder and arm that had previously been excessive, disappeared in five minutes; the hand was then drawn down the injured part for three or four minutes, and he experienced more ease than he had for the previous month, a little soreness on the part near the nail being only left. He immediately threw the leather into the fire-place and removed the cerate which was ordered by the surgeon. He was then enabled to do many things

which he had not done for the previous month. This gentleman, who he believes was Mr. Capern of Devonshire, visited him the next morning, and, the hand being again drawn over the thumb, the soreness disappeared, and he is now, thanks to Mr. Capern, able to attend to his customary duties. He slept better the night after the operation than he had done for the previous month. Mr. Byron, of Byron's Tavern, may be referred to.

George Wood.

4. Copy of a letter received from Joseph Dowton, in the employ of Mr. George Cosway, woollen manufacturer, Tiverton.

"Tiverton, Nov. 21st, 1849.

"To Mr. Thomas Capern.

"For six months I was suffering most excruciating pain in my head, caused by that dreadful complaint, tic douloureux. I tried a great many things to relieve the pain, but nothing I used had the least effect. By the kind persuasions of some friends, I made application to you; and through that invaluable science, mesmerism, and through the passes which you made round and about my head, it entirely removed the pain, and I have never felt it since, for which kind act and the power of your valuable science I shall ever feel grateful.

"Believe me ever to remain, dear sir,

"Under the greatest obligation,

"Joseph Dowton."

5. Janeretta Tout, aged 45 years, wife of James Tout, agricultural labourer, Manley, Tiverton, states

that she had the tic douloureux in the head for nearly sixteen years. She consulted, at various times, eleven surgeons and two physicians, and was for seventeen days an in-patient of Barnstaple Hospital; but without the least benefit. Instead of becoming better, she grew worse and worse, the attacks lasting sometimes twelve or thirteen hours, and the pain being extremely severe. In September, 1849, (a little more than three months since) she was induced to apply to Mr. Capern to be mesmerised. There was an immediate improvement after the first operation. She has been mesmerised about six or seven times since, and each time with increased benefit. She seldom suffers any pain now, except when something happens that irritates and makes her anxious. The pain, when it does occur, is much less severe now than formerly, and lasts a shorter time. She was also subject for many years to soreness of the breast; this complaint has been much better since she applied to Mr. Capern. Some years ago she met with an accident and injured her left arm and shoulder. She subsequently suffered from rheumatism in the same part, and for the last three years she has been unable to put her left hand behind her. Until this day (5th January) she had never mentioned it to Mr. Capern, who had therefore almost entirely confined his passes to the head. A rock-crystal being drawn down the arm, not with any intention of benefiting the limb, but merely by way of experiment, a strong sensation of warmth was produced, and in a few minutes she was able to place her hand quite behind her, and move the fingers and arm with greater ease and freedom. She also experienced powerful effects from the rock-crystal being placed opposite her eyes for a few minutes. A strong sensation of warmth in the temples, with a feeling of greater lightness and comfort took place. At this first mesmerisation she swooned completely away, and on every subsequent occasion she experienced great faintness, and it was necessary to support her in the chair, or she would most certainly have fallen to the ground.

Tiverton, January, 1850.

6. [Certificate.] "I, Benjamin Wood, do hereby testify that in 1847 I was taken with a seizure in my right foot and leg, as though my ankle was disjointed. I went to Mr. Capern, who made some passes over the part affected, and made a complete cure of it. In 1848 I was taken with a lumbago in my back, when I was again operated upon by Mr. Capern with similar success. In the beginning of this year (1849) I was seized with a very violent pain in my head, which continued for a long time; so that I was obliged to apply to a doctor; but after trying various means, and finding no relief, I was again obliged to go to Mr. Capern, and by his operations I received a perfect cure of that painful disease, the tic douloureux.

"BENJAMIN WOOD."

7. Mrs. DRANE, Bampton Street, Tiverton, states as follows :—"I had confirmed tic douloureux in the head for upwards of five years, so bad that I have been confined to my bed six months at a time, with three sur-

geons attending me at once, and at last they pronounced me incurable. I have had a gallon of water night and morning thrown over my head, it being so excessively hot. I applied to Mr. Capern, and after the passes had been frequently made by him on me, I am quite recovered."

8. Sarah Lee, St. Andrew's Street, Tiverton, aged 54 years, states that nearly three years since she had an attack of tic douloureux of a very severe character for several weeks, during a portion of which time she could not rest her head on the pillow. She was induced to name it to Mr. Capern, who commenced operating upon her. After the passes had been made for a few minutes, a sensation of heat was produced and relief afforded. At the second operation she was completely cured, and continued well until Christmas 1849, when she took a chill, which was followed by a return of the disease. After four sittings, however, the pains entirely disappeared.

9. John Lee, Hammett's Lane, shoemaker, had a severe attack of tic douloureux, about eighteen months since, so that for a fortnight he could not do any work and had little or no rest. He also totally lost his appetite, and, although many remedies were applied, no good effect resulted. He then applied to Mr. Capern, and immediately after the passes were made over him the pains left him. Above five months since he had another attack. He applied to Mr. C. again. The pains were entirely subdued and he has had no return of them since.

He had been advised to apply to Mr. Capern day after day to be mesmerised, but had refused on the ground that he had no faith whatever in mesmerism.

10. Copy of a letter received from Mr. William Goodland.

"Tiverton, May 4th, 1850.

"Dear Sir,—I beg very respectfully to give my testimony to the fact of having received a perfect cure, by means of mesmerism, from the most distressing affliction that falls to the lot of a human being to suffer, viz. tic douloureux of the most excruciating kind. For many years I resided in Bristol, and during six of those years the above-named disease was gradually making progress, notwithstanding my having procured the best medical advice in the city. My case was pronounced incurable, and nothing could relieve me of my painful malady. My family and myself much feared that ultimately it would terminate in lock-jaw. But, however, a kind Providence interfered, and I was removed from Bristol to this place, and applied to you when in pain; and after the head and face had been mesmerised for three months, I am happy to say, as I said at the commencement of my letter, that I am perfectly restored to health, and for several months past have not experienced the slightest relapse.

"I remain, dear sir,

"Yours very affectionately,

"WILLIAM GOODLAND.

"Mr. T. Capern."

11. Mrs. Susan Hawkins, of Water Lane, Tiverton, suffered from most severe tic douloureux in the back of the head, temples, forehead, and both jaws, for seven years. During this period she was under the treatment of many medical men, civil and military, her husband being a soldier. But nothing that was done ever procured her the slightest relief. Her sufferings at last were most excruciating, rendering her quite incapable of paying any attention to, or doing, anything for her family. The attacks came on regularly every day. Her forehead and eyes would swell to a fearful extent, and she would become nearly blind as long as the attacks lasted. Deriving no relief from the ordinary practitioners, she had recourse to quack medicines, upon which she spent a great many pounds; but without any beneficial results. A friend of hers recommended her to apply to Mr. Capern. She followed this advice, and, being unable to walk alone, she was assisted by two of her neighbours to his house. After Mr. Capern had mesmerised her for a few minutes she experienced immediate relief. At the third operation she felt a great ringing in the ears and a loud noise in the head, like the report of a pistol. She continued under the mesmeric treatment for about a month; at the end of which time she was perfectly cured, and she has since remained quite well although three years have elapsed. No person in Tiverton now questions her statement, though, at the period when the cure was made, she would not have been believed upon her oath, and was frequently jeered and scoffed at on mentioning her case.

12. WILLIAM BURTON, Tuspot House, Bampton Down, aged 74 years. In August, 1849, met with a severe accident, by which his right leg was fractured. It was five o'clock on a Monday afternoon when the accident occurred, and until the afternoon of Wednesday in the same week he was in constant pain. His sufferings were very severe, without any interval of ease, and he could obtain no rest whatever. On Wednesday afternoon Mr. Capern operated upon the limb with non-contact passes for about seven or eight minutes. Immediate relief was the result, and from that time he enjoyed perfect ease; the pain never once returning, even in the slightest degree. Some time before the accident he had suffered from hydrocele, which occasioned severe pain in the part. After the accident the pain became constant, and very much increased in severity, but after Mr. Capern had operated upon him it entirely ceased, and he has never been troubled with it since. At a somewhat later period sores also appeared round or about the ankle of the injured limb, but they never caused him the least pain even when they were dressed.

13. JOHN CROOTE states that his wife, Elizabeth Croote, had a seizure after her confinement, which took place sixteen years ago, and from that time she was never able to attend to her domestic affairs. For the last three years she was wholly confined to her bed, and was not, during that period, able to sit up. Mr. Capern, having called and seen her in that lamentable condition, offered to operate upon her. The effect produced was unexpected by Mr. Capern. After a few

passes she slept well and was relieved from pain. After a few mesmerisations the improvement was so extraordinary that she was able, whilst in bed, to sit and make several garments, which she had not been able to do for many years.

14. MARY GROGAN, Bickleigh, aged 33 years, states that she had the milk fever after her confinement. The pains were very severe in the knee, and then removed to the hand, which prevented her from working. She applied to a surgeon in the neighbourhood and a physician in Exeter. The pains were slightly mitigated for a time, but then appeared again, as badly as before. She applied to Mr. Capern, and was immediately better than she had been for six months previous. After three sittings she was cured.

15. WILLIAM ISAACS, carpenter, West-Exe, Tiverton, in the employ of John Heathcoat, Esq., M.P., was suddenly seized in the autumn of 1847, while employed at the bench, with severe pains in the groin, and which immediately afterwards extended to the foot. The pain near the knee was excruciating. He thought at first it was caused by a splinter; but on examination it was proved that this was not the case. He was carried home by two men and put to bed, and two surgeons were immediately called in, who advised his removal to the hospital. The agonies he endured were fearful. On one occasion, an attempt being made to remove him in his bed, he fainted with the pain. The leg and foot were enormously swelled—so much so, that

when he extended his leg straight before him he was unable to see his toes. This continued several weeks. The surgeon believing that there was a formation of matter, made an incision in the limb near the knee. A small quantity of matter then issued from the wound, but the operation afforded him no relief whatever. He was confined to his bed for nearly two months, during which time the pain was most excruciating. He had no rest whatever: he was nearly worn out for want of sleep: his appetite was gone, and he was reduced to a state of great weakness, despairing of obtaining any relief from the surgeons. Being strongly advised by his friends, he applied to Mr. Capern. He procured a pair of new crutches and left his home for the purpose of going to Mr. C.'s residence. He was unable to put his foot to the ground, and it was only with great difficulty that he could manage to get along. Happening to meet Mr. Capern on Exe Bridge he stated his object. Mr. C. invited him to turn back and accompany him to the Swan Inn (not far from his own house). At the very first pass he experienced some relief; and in less than five minutes he was entirely free from pain. He was so delighted and astonished at his sudden and unexpected cure, that he hardly knew what he was about; and without even waiting to thank Mr. C., shouldered his crutches, and ran off to the workshop, where he made his appearance, to the great amazement of his fellow workmen, who knew the state to which he had been reduced. From the workshop he proceeded to the club-house, where he gave notice of his intention to relinquish his sick-pay. This was on a Friday, and on the following Monday he was in full work. He has never had a return of the pain, or lost a day's work since. At the time of his application to Mr. Capern he had no faith whatever in mesmerism.

16. "This is to certify that my wife was suffering the most excruciating pain in her head and face from tic douloureux. She could take no rest, nor scarcely eat any food. She tried various things to no purpose. I advised her to call on Mr. Thos. Capern. She did; so he made a few passes of the hand over the face, and in less than two minutes the pain was gone. This was done in August last.

"H. T. Risdon.

"Tiverton, Devon.

"January 15th, 1851."

SECTION III.

TOOTHACHE.

1. BESSY STEPHENS, daughter of James Stephens, of Bampton Street, Tiverton, painter, &c., had suffered for three weeks from severe pains in the face, supposed to be toothache. The tooth was taken out; but there was no mitigation of the pain, which was then declared by the operator to proceed from rheumatism. She was in great agony, and cried and moaned almost without intermission from Saturday evening till Tuesday afternoon. Her father was so affected by her sufferings that he left the house, unable any longer to be witness of them. He bent his steps towards Mr. Capern's house, with the view of requesting his assistance. Mr. C. returned with him, and put the girl into the mesmeric sleep; but she still continued crying and moaning, and was awake in half an hour with the pain as great as ever. Mr. C. commenced making contact passes down the face and arm. After a few passes, the pain moved downward, following the direction of his fingers; a few more and it was in the arm near the shoulder; a few more and it was in the fore arm and wrist, and then in the fingers, which suddenly became quite rigid; a few more and the pain had entirely disappeared. The whole process did not occupy more than five minutes.

This patient died of consumption about twelve months

afterwards; but during the whole of that period the pain never once returned.

NOTE.—The above case is important, inasmuch as it demonstrates the efficacy of the mesmeric "passes" in a case where the mere production of the "sleep" seemed of little avail.

2. SARAH MANNING, Townsend, Tiverton, 37 years, suffered severe pains in the teeth and jaws from her childhood; and for the last twelve years the pain has been so violent that at times she has been almost deprived of her senses. She applied to Mr. Capern about three years since, and, after a few operations, experienced more ease and comfort than she had during that period. She has had no return of the pain since.

January 4th, 1850.

3. SARAH HOARE, aged 30 years, had suffered for three years and a half from severe toothache. During the whole of that time she had never passed a single week free from pain. At times it was most excruciating, and when Mr. Capern first saw her she was in great agony. By a few mesmeric passes on her face she was released from all the pain for the time; but it returned, though very slightly, some time after the operation, and she felt her head very hot during the whole of the night. She was mesmerised three times afterwards, and she now scarcely ever suffers toothache, and never severely.

4. Statement of CHARLOTTE MORRELL, West Barton, Tiverton.

"I had severe toothache for seven months. Mr. Capern came to my house to enquire after my father, whom he had cured of rheumatism. I stated my case to him, and he immediately made the passes over my face. The pain instantly left me, and since then I have never had a return of it. This occurred about three years ago."

September 20th, 1849.

5. JOHN VICKERY, hairdresser, West Exe, Tiverton, had suffered, for about five years, from severe toothache, which frequently rendered him incapable of attending to his occupation, and he often passed several nights in succession without any sleep. Various attempts had been made by different surgeons to extract the teeth, but they all failed. Having heard that Mr. Capern had cured a case of toothache, he was induced to apply to that gentleman, and, meeting him accidentally in the street, while in a state of great suffering, Mr. C. took him into the shop of Mr. Wellington, a druggist, and in his presence, in about two or three minutes, relieved him from all pain, and completely cured the toothache by merely looking at him at the distance of about three feet. This occurred nearly three years ago, and he has not had the slightest return of it. Mr. Capern, having heard of cures being made by mesmerists by the mere will, and without passes, was desirous of making the experiment for the purpose of ascertaining the fact, and from the success of this experiment is convinced that with sensitive patients a cure may often be performed in this way.

6. "I, George Greenslade, labourer, in the employ of John Heathcoat, Esq., M.P., Tiverton, do hereby certify that I was suffering from a pain in the teeth and jaw for three weeks, a fortnight of which time the pains were so violent that I could have knocked my head against a wall. For the great part of two days and one night I took no food whatever. I was induced to apply to Mr. Capern, who requested me to sit opposite to him and look him steadfastly in the face; I did so, and within the space of two minutes I felt a shock all over my body, and in about three minutes afterwards the pain moved from the jaw to the back part of the head, afterwards returned to the jaw, and in three minutes more it was entirely gone; and I was enabled to resume my labour with ease. A pass was not made over me by Mr. Capern.

"Tiverton, August 10th, 1850."

The mark of George ⋈ Greenslade.

The above cure took place in the presence of J. Cross, Esq., artist, of London, who witnessed the extraordinary effect produced over the body. It appeared like an electric shock.

John Cross.

SECTION IV.

SPRAINS.

1. Betsy Isaacs, wife of William Isaacs, lives in West Exe, Tiverton. Was taken giddy about seven weeks ago, and losing her sight fell down; the left leg turned under her and the ankle became strained, so that she could scarcely move the foot, and in getting up stairs had to go upon her knee for several days for the first fortnight, and suffered a great deal of pain. She met Mr. Capern in the street on the 10th June, being in pain and limping from the state of her ancle, and requested Mr. Capern to try if he could help her. He accordingly accompanied her to a neighbouring house, and commenced making passes down the knee and ankle. She declared she felt a change at the second pass, and in three minutes afterwards that the pain had entirely ceased. She then walked across the room with the greatest ease.

Mr. Capern had, about three months previously, relieved her of a severe toothache.

Betsy Isaacs, ⋈ her mark.

2. Mrs. Sarah Lee, of St. Andrews Street, Tiverton, states that her son John Lee, now aged 18 years, was brought home to her house with a severe sprain in the ankle. He was confined to his bed for six days;

at the end of which time he gained sufficient strength to walk with the assistance of a crutch and stick. He accidentally met Mr. Capern in Fore Street, who hearing his case invited him into a house, and after a few passes over the limb he dispensed with his crutch and on the following day walked without either crutch or stick. From that time he has been free from pain.

3. Thomas Howard, mason, Tiverton, in the employ of Mr. Beck, fell from the roof of a house, and received considerable injury in the back and shoulders. He was assisted home, and when placed in bed had no power of motion, and suffered extreme pain. Mr. Capern was requested to operate on him, and consented; and after making a few passes with the hand over the affected part the first sensation was a comfortable glow of heat, and then the patient was able to lie down on the bed. From that time his sleep was improved. He was operated upon once or twice a day for seven or eight days, and each successive time felt the effects of the passes. Since the last mesmerisation he has been able to labour as well as he did before the accident.

4. James Wreford, painter and carpenter, Stockleigh Pomeroy, states that in the month of December, 1848 he fell on the ice and sprained his wrist. After trying various remedies without benefit, he consulted a professional gentleman in Exeter with the same result. He then applied to Mr. Capern, and was completely cured by three applications of the mesmeric power.

5. THOMAS COSWAY, hairdresser, West Exe, Tiverton, had a severe fall about ten years ago, and injured his hand and wrist, from which accident he suffered much pain and inconvenience until between two and three years ago, when, happening to meet Mr. Capern, and hearing him converse about mesmerism and the cure of rheumatism, he said to Mr. C. in a joking, bantering way, he had a bad pain in his wrist, and asked him to cure that. Mr. C. made a few passes on his wrist, and he derived immediate benefit. He was operated upon four or five times afterwards, and completely relieved from all pain.

January 4, 1850.

6. HENRY FOWLER, aged 5 years, when about two years old severely sprained his ankle. He was unable to walk or even to put his foot to the ground; the limb was much swollen as far as the knee, and the swelling was gradually extending itself. No medical aid was called in; but the child's mother bathed the affected part frequently in a mixture of warm water and bran, and a bandage was constantly worn round it. Under this treatment there was no improvement whatever. About a fortnight after the accident, Mr. Capern happened to see the child in the arms of the woman who had charge of him. Having been informed of the child's state, he made a few passes over the limb. This occurred in the forenoon. When the child's mother returned home to dinner, she found to her great surprise that he was able to walk. The limb was not bathed any more, and the bandage was removed. The child

continued to improve, and in about a week he was quite well, the swelling of the limb having completely disappeared. Mr. Capern did not see the child after the operation, and had quite forgotten the circumstance, until he was reminded of it by his little patient's mother, who a few days ago brought another of her children to be operated upon.

SECTION V.

PARALYSIS, &c.

1. HARRIET HARRIS, Townsend, Tiverton, suffered from paralysis, brought on by hooping-cough, also from extreme enervation and weakness, to such a degree that she could not carry a jug or light weight across the house with safety. She felt great relief shortly after the passes were made. She continued to improve, and is now completely cured.

2. WILLIAM MANLEY, mason, Tiverton, aged 64 years, states as follows:—That in the summer of 1848, whilst walking in Fore Street, he was seized with a fit of apoplexy, was carried home, and remained in a state of insensibility for eight days. On his return to consciousness he found his left side paralysed. He was attended by four surgeons, and at the end of four weeks was sufficiently recovered to be able to walk with the assistance of a stick. But his left arm hung paralysed and useless by his side. Having occasion to visit a relation, who kept a public house called the Barrington Bell, in Tiverton, and being seated at the fireside in the parlour, Mr. Capern entered, having occasion to transact some business, and seated himself near the place where he was sitting. He did not observe that Mr. C. had placed his hand on his shoulder, until he became

very warm and faint. He then turned round and said, "Good God! what are you doing to me?" Mr. C. desired him to remain quiet, and said that he was glad to hear that he had those sensations, as he thought he should be able to do him some good. After having made a few passes upon his arm Mr. Capern left him; but Manley was in so profuse a perspiration that he was unable to leave the house for a full hour. Subsequently Mr. C. operated upon him every day, for about three months, when he was quite cured, having the full use of both arms and able to resume his labour. During the last few weeks of the mesmeric operations, and even at the present day, Mr. C. could throw him into a state of profuse perspiration, by merely looking at him steadfastly for a few minutes. He was never put into a state of coma, but his feet have been fixed on the floor by one or two passes.

3. Copy of a letter received from Mr. William Goodland, Tiverton.

"Peter's Street, 14th May, 1849.

"I respectfully beg to give my testimony to the public, that my wife has been most powerfully relieved in consequence of the means used by Mr. Thomas Capern. She had been paralysed for nearly fourteen years, during which period she suffered much from confusion of the head, so that at times she was almost lost to the things and persons around her. She was scarcely able to take a cup from the table with safety, so weak was her hand. Now she can take a small copper tea-kettle from the fire and fill the teapot. Also she experienced great difficulty in going up and down stairs, and was fearful of placing her weak foot first. Now she can place it in an ordinary way as well as myself, and without being afraid of falling. She also can take a walk alone a distance of three or four miles; whereas before, if she went outside of the door without some one assisting her, she was afraid to walk, thinking that every one she met was going to push her down. She consulted several eminent surgeons in Bristol, but without receiving any benefit. I could say much, much more; but what I have already said I hope will suffice.

"WILLIAM GOODLAND."

4. DAN FOWLER, West Exe, Tiverton, 5 months old, November 2nd, 1850. When born, his left arm was utterly useless and hung behind his back. Three days after his birth his grandmother went to a medical man, who considered that a muscle was deficient. A month afterwards the mother applied to this gentleman. He said nothing could be done until the child was three months old; but suggested that salt and water should be used. The same day she consulted Mr. Capern, who then for the first time mesmerised the child. Great moisture was produced along the course of the arm, and particularly at the finger's end; this was in July. Mr. C. continued his operations daily for three months. During two months the child always cried, but after that he looked up and laughed whilst being operated upon. About the end of the first month, the mother began to observe the fingers move, and gradually the

entire arm; then the child commenced to seize the articles within his reach and to raise the arm up.

The presumed cause of the child's condition was the circumstance of a brother of Dan having been drowned, and the first part of the body seen by the mother being its left arm, which caused a great fright. The mother gave birth to Dan about four months afterwards. At birth the left arm was much smaller, at present it is much larger, than the other. During the last two months the child has been gradually getting better; and each time the operation is performed there is an increase of warmth in the limb.

5. Copy of a letter received from H. Colquhoun, Esq.

"Tiverton, May 3rd, 1850.

"Dear Sir,—My son George Arthur being now cured of his troublesome complaint, viz., non-retention of urine at night (he will be 7 years of age next birthday), I think it but just that mesmerism should have my testimony as to this cure. This boy had previously been under medical treatment by the most eminent physicians and surgeons in London. On my return from India, I found his complaint most offensive; and, after sea-bathing, tonics, and sleeping on hard mattrasses had failed, I had recourse to you, knowing, from what I have seen in India of mesmerism under Dr. Esdaile, that the system would be strengthened, even if a cure were not effected. The result has been in my opinion a perfect cure, no return of the complaint having occurred for three months; and this without medicine or any attention to diet in particular except mesmerised water. Pray accept my sincere thanks for the trouble you have had. The cure was effected in seventeen days, you operating once for half-an-hour daily.

"I remain, dear sir,

"Yours faithfully and truly,

"H. COLQUHOUN.

"Mr. Thos. Capern."

SECTION VI.

HEADACHE, NOISES IN THE HEAD, &c.

1. Statement received from Mrs. Wilson, Fore Street, Tiverton.

"Harriet Cornish, when in a mesmeric sleep, told me, in answer to Mr. Capern, that my complaint was entirely in the nerves, that no medicine would do me any good, but that Mr. C. could cure me by making passes, which she described. She also told me I was suffering severely in the face and head; that the pain which I felt in my ears was occasioned by the weakness of the nerves; and that there was something in Mr. Beedell's shop which would effect a cure if I would send for a pennyworth; that this 'something' was in a small bottle on the fourth shelf, on the left hand side on going into the parlour, and was the fourth bottle; that there were three other bottles of the same in different parts of the shop, and that they were not marked. I was to drop one drop on a little bit of wadding, and put in each ear; then wrap my face in flannel, which would be the better if Mr. C. would mesmerise it; and to drink, as soon as I awoke, mesmerised water, which would strengthen me. I sent for the drug according to her description, and applied it with success, being much relieved within five minutes. I have now been under Mr. Capern's care for a fortnight; and with feelings of the deepest gratitude I confess the effects of his passes have been almost miraculous on me. As mine was entirely a disorder of the nervous system, medical advice was of no avail; whereas the mesmeric passes have sustained me, I may say with comfort, through a time of great trial and vexation, the contemplation of which at times nearly disordered my intellects. I am much stronger both in body and mind; and my only regret at leaving Tiverton is, that I shall be deprived of Mr. Capern's kind attention. I take this opportunity of assuring that gentleman that I shall always feel the deepest gratitude towards him; as I am well assured that he has been the means, under a merciful Providence, of saving my life.

"EMMA WILSON.

"Tiverton, Sept. 29th, 1849."

2. MARY TAYLOR, West Exe, Tiverton, aged 54 years, had been subject to severe headaches ever since she was ten years old. For some time previous to her applying to Mr. Capern, a week never passed without their occurring two or three times. They usually lasted twenty-four hours; during one half of which time she was very sick. She was reduced to a state of great weakness; and was almost entirely disabled from performing any household work. As soon as the attacks came on, she was completely prostrated, and when in service was often (to use her own expression) carried to bed like a dead person. She slept little, and never knew what it was to awake in the morning without a pain in the head. About two years ago, she was in-

duced to apply to Mr. Capern, by whom she was mesmerised about forty times. She has derived great benefit from the mesmeric treatment. She does not now suffer from headache more than once in three or four months. At the present time she has been six or seven months free from an attack. When they do occur they are of short duration, and less severe than formerly, seldom lasting more than eleven or twelve hours. The household occupations, for which she was formerly obliged to employ a person, she now performs with her own hands. She sleeps well. During the last two years she has several times sat up as a nurse with sick persons, and on one occasion for ten successive nights. On two other occasions for eight nights, and on a fourth for six nights; and only on the first of those occasions did she suffer from headache, and even then the attack did not come on until the last morning, when she was obliged to return home. She declares that she has not been so well as she now is, since she was a little girl ten years of age.

3. Mrs. COOKSLEY, Hammett's Lane, suffered extreme pain in the head for three years; which, at times, prevented her from attending to her domestic affairs. She applied to surgeons, who afforded no relief. After the passes had been made over her three or four times by Mr. Capern she was quite restored.

4. MARY LAND, of Bampton Street, aged about 70, was afflicted for many years (she thinks about fifteen), with dreadful noises in the head, attended with pain,

which rendered existence completely miserable. She states that it is impossible to describe the noises, as they were entirely different from any thing she has ever heard in her life. Although she was never wholly free from them at any time, they occurred with increased violence when she was in bed, and were always worse every other night. The terror and distraction which they occasioned were often so extreme that she would scream at intervals the whole night through, and so loudly that the policemen on duty have come in to enquire what was the matter. She declares that on these occasions nothing whatever,—no threat, not even of instant death, could have kept her quiet. Her nights were almost sleepless, and every other night she was certain to get no rest whatever. At times she was unable to remain in her bed from the dreadful annoyance caused by the noises, but was obliged to get up and walk about the room, even during the coldest nights in winter. She speaks of her sufferings as being extreme. She knew not what it was to enjoy ease and comfort, or to be a moment free from anxiety; since she was never safe from an attack, and never knew when the noises might come on with violence. Her mind was so much affected that the parish authorities had it in view to send her to a lunatic asylum. Her memory was also greatly impaired, so that during the period of her illness she was unable to keep an exact account of time, and cannot state with any degree of certainty what was the duration of her sufferings. She was incapable of occupying herself with reading, of which she had previously been very fond. She consulted three physicians and three surgeons, but without the least benefit. She believed that it would have been impossible for her to have borne her sufferings much longer, and that very soon she must either have gone mad, or sunk under them and died. Shortly before the noises came on she had rheumatic and nervous fever, and had also been subject to tic douloureux. At length she was advised by a friend to apply to Mr. Capern, but was very reluctant to do so. Nevertheless, Mr. Capern went to see her, and commenced operating upon her daily. For three weeks no effects resulted from the treatment. She frequently urged him not to trouble himself any more about her, as she felt persuaded that all his exertions for her relief would be in vain. After three weeks she felt something which she called a "creeping sensation" in her head when the passes were made over it. The violent attacks began to occur less frequently and to diminish in intensity. The improvement was slow and gradual. For three months she was mesmerised daily, and afterwards less frequently for some time longer. She now considers herself cured, for though she is still subject to an almost constant singing in the ears, this, in comparison with the old noises, she looks upon as only a trifling inconvenience. Her life is comfortable and easy, and she is again able to employ herself in reading. She speaks of her recovery and Mr. Capern's kind attention in the warmest terms of gratitude.

October, 1849.

SECTION VII.

EPILEPSY.

Leah Wood, West Exe, Tiverton, aged 15 years, was subject to epileptic fits from her ninth year. They sometimes occurred as often as four or five times a week; and she was never, at any time, free from them longer than a fortnight. Her mother was afraid to trust her away from home alone, as the attacks were liable to come on without any previous warning. They sometimes lasted twenty-four hours; during which time she remained in a state of unconsciousness, laughing and talking, and sometimes struggling so violently as to require two or three men to hold her. She had become, in consequence, very weak and emaciated, her intellect much impaired, her countenance vacant, and her appearance altogether idiotic and silly. The boys frequently followed her in the streets hooting and mocking. About three years ago Mr. Capern commenced mesmerising her, and continued to do so for upwards of a year and a half. She derived great benefit from his operations: the fits occurring much less frequently—not oftener than once in six months, and even then they were generally brought on by some strong excitement—as for instance, about six or seven months ago, when sent to service against her inclination. They are also altered in character. On the occasion just alluded to there was no laughing or talking, but she remained almost entirely motionless during the whole time, not opening her lips once from 9 p.m. till 11 a.m. next day. Her appearance and her intellects are much improved as well as her general health, and she is now able to be of some use to her mother in her house, though she is still very nervous, and everything calculated to cause excitement is necessarily avoided. Several weeks elapsed before Mr. Capern could induce sleep in this case, and when he at length succeeded, it was accompanied by a peculiar motion of the head, hands, and right leg, which moved from side to side whilst she remained in the sleep-waking state. Her mesmerist, however, shortly discovered that, by placing one finger on the organ of Firmness, and another on one of the vertebræ of the neck, he had the power of arresting these motions. After being under treatment for some months, his patient whilst in the sleep-waking state informed him that by making certain passes, which she proceeded to describe, he could effectually and permanently stop these motions; he did so, and they have never once occurred since. This patient remains very susceptible of the mesmeric influence, and is put into a state of coma at any time, in two or three seconds, by the mere will of her mesmeriser. She is also a tolerably good clairvoyante.

SECTION VIII.

ST. VITUS'S DANCE.

John Rooks, aged 14 years, Martin's Lane, Tiverton, had St. Vitus's dance for seven weeks, in consequence of an injury received from falling forward, by which his whole weight was thrown upon his thumb. His parents applied to a surgeon and a physician, by both of whom the disease was declared to be Chorea or Vitus's dance. The medicine which was given him produced no beneficial effect, and was discontinued as soon as the mesmeric treatment commenced. He was mesmerised daily by Mr. Capern for the first three weeks, and afterwards less frequently. A complete cure was effected in seven or eight weeks.

SECTION IX.

INFLAMMATIONS, &c.

1. STATEMENT received from Mr. John Rogers, of Barnstaple Gate, Tiverton.

"Dec. 26th, 1849.

"I had an inflammation in the right leg from the knee down to the foot for above six weeks, during which time I had no comfortable rest. I applied various remedies as suggested by different persons without any improvement, until one morning about six o'clock Mr. Capern passing the house, and observing that I was in pain, enquired the cause; on my relating it to him, he came into the house, and, after his passing the hand over the part for a few minutes, I had relief, and from that time an improvement took place. In about twelve days all pain had gone and I am now as well as I ever was.

"From JOHN ROGERS.

"Mr. Capern, Tiverton, Devon."

2. Copy of a letter received from Mr. John Rutley to Mr. Thomas Capern.

"Sir,—It is with much pleasure I return you my sincere thanks for the kindness and great benefit I received from you during my short visit at Tiverton.

In the month of March 1844, I was afflicted with scrofula in the right knee-joint. I became an in-patient of the Bath United hospital, where I remained for three months under the care of that celebrated surgeon, George Norman, Esq. He wanted to amputate the limb, but to this I would not consent: so he very unceremoniously ordered me to leave the hospital immediately. I accordingly left it and sent for an herbalist, and to the virtue of herbs, under God's blessing, I attribute the salvation not only of my limb, but of my life also. I remained under the care of this herbalist for ten weeks, when I was able again to resume my usual employment. About fourteen months afterwards it got rather worse than usual: so I consulted a surgeon from Ireland, and was under his care about fourteen weeks and found great benefit from his treatment of the case. About twelvemonths after this my knee got worse again: so I became an in-patient of the Bristol infirmary, where I was treated with great kindness and care; but the only benefit I found was from the rest I got. A month after this I returned to Tiverton, and on my arrival found that a neighbour of mine had found great benefit in mesmerism. This induced me, Sir, to call on you; and the mesmerism with the tartar emetic ointment has benefited me more than any remedy previously tried; and I firmly believe that if I could have remained in Tiverton three months longer, under the care of Messrs. Parker and Capern, I should have received a perfect cure, although the case is a very obstinate one of long standing. I am greatly indebted to you, Mr. Capern, for your kindness, and to Mr. Parker, of Exeter; if you see him, please to thank him for me. I really wish every surgeon in England would add mesmerism to their practice, I am sure they would if they had personally felt the great benefit from it that I have.

"JOHN RUTLEY.

"21, Castle Green, Bristol.
"Oct. 28th, 1847."

"P.S. I omitted to say that for the last eight days I have walked a distance of fifteen miles per day: an undertaking which for the last five years I have been unable until now to perform."

3. MARY ANN ARTHUR, of Stoodleigh, states that she was suffering for four months from a severe inflammation of the right knee, during the greater part of which time she was incapable of attending to her regular employment, and it was with the greatest difficulty she could walk. She applied to surgeons at Bampton and Tiverton, but without being at all benefited by them. She was induced by some friends of hers, residing at Oakford, to apply to Mr. Capern: which she did. At the first application she felt less pain; and after the third she was completely cured. This took place in the summer of 1849, and she has had no pain from that time.

Huntland, March 10th, 1850.

4. JAMES GILL, painter and glazier, was subject for many years to severe attacks of inflammation of the heels. During the hot weather of summer he was sel-

dom free from the complaint. In the year 1847 the attack was more severe than usual. The pain was for three weeks excruciating. His heels were much inflamed, and of a deep red color, (like "raw beef," to use his mother's expression): and he was quite unable to place them upon the ground. Mr. Capern, being sent for, attended, and made the usual passes over the affected parts. Very great relief was felt from the first operation. Next day he was mesmerised a second time: and on the day following he went to Bampton, a distance of seven miles to his work, calling on his way at Mr. Capern's to receive a few passes. He has remained quite free from the pain ever since.

5. MRS. WOODMAN, Bampton Street, had inflammatory affection of the head for three years, so that at times when she got out of bed she was unable to move about for more than an hour. After the passes had been made a few times she became relieved, and in a short time she was as well as ever.

6. JAMES KING, tea-dealer, Tiverton, received a blow in the neck about eight years ago, which caused the glands to swell, and he experienced very great pains in consequence. He applied to surgeons and physicians in Tiverton, Exeter, Teignmouth, and Plymouth, and was under medical treatment for eight years. From one surgeon alone he took no less than eighteen quart bottles of medicine. But neither these nor anything that was done for him by the doctors were of the slightest

service. His neck had become frightfully diseased, there being as many as eighteen open wounds in it at a time: as fast as one wound suppurated another formed, and there was a constant discharge of large quantities of matter. He happened to be present when Mrs. Teesdale was in a state of sleep-waking, and she called Mr. Capern's attention to King's affliction, and informed him that he might cure King by mesmerism, at the same time giving directions in what manner the passes were to be made. At the end of about twenty applications of about five minutes duration each the wounds closed and were perfectly healed, and they have remained so ever since.

7. William Browning, aged five months. Three days after the birth of this child a discharge of matter commenced from the ears. This discharge, so copious as to saturate the child's cap, continued uninterruptedly for sixteen weeks; and when Mr. Capern commenced his operations about a month ago there was an immediate improvement, and as the operations were continued the discharge became less and less. It has now entirely ceased.

July 4th, 1850.

8. Martha Short, Frog Street, Tiverton, states that after her confinement she had a violent pain in the breast, which was relieved by a few passes made by Mr. Capern. The same evening as she was operated upon the breast suppurated, and discharged a quantity

of matter. The mesmeric passes being repeated, the breast, after a few sittings, was completely cured.

The nurse that attended her states that she never saw a cure so rapidly effected. This took place two years since, and she has been well from that time.

October 29th, 1849.

SECTION X.

AFFECTIONS OF THE EYES.

1. Copy of a letter from Sarah Ann Mogford, Stoodleigh.

"November 27th, 1849.

"Sir,—From a deep sense of gratitude I feel bound to return my sincere thanks for the benefit I have experienced at your hands. I was afflicted with dimness of sight for seven or eight years before I applied to you, and through your kind attention to my case I am happy to say that the organs of vision are restored. I have only again to thank you for your kindness and attention.

"I remain, gratefully, Sir,

"Your humble servant,

"Sarah Ann Mogford.

"To Mr. Thomas Capern, Tiverton."

2. Mrs. Ann Fulford, East Anstey, states that she had weak eyes for upwards of eight years; and within the last twelve months they became worse; so much so that she could not read large print, and calculated upon a total privation of sight. Having been informed that Mr. Capern had afforded relief to several persons, she was induced to apply to him, when he made some passes over her eyes. A little improvement

took place. After six sittings her sight was perfectly restored.

N.B. East Anstey is twelve miles from Tiverton, and she had to leave her family for a whole day to have the benefit of the passes.

3. Copy of a letter from Mr. William Skinner, Thorverton.

"July 6th, 1849.

"Sir,—In answer to your letter dated the 4th instant, I write to inform you of the state of my eyes previously to my going to the Eye Infirmary. First of all there was something over them so that I could scarcely see anything. The surgeons told me it was a cataract, and that I should have to go through an operation. In about a month afterwards they told me it was something else. I attended the infirmary several times for ten or twelve weeks, without deriving any benefit. At last I was recommended to apply to you; which I did, and derived great benefit from your treatment. I think I came to you eight or nine times; and, thank God, I can now see almost as well as ever I could. In returning my sincere and hearty thanks,

"I am, Sir, your most obliged servant,

"WILLIAM SKINNER.

"To Mr. Capern."

4. JAMES HILL, son of William Hill, East Anstey, aged 4 years, was suddenly attacked about one month ago with inflammation of both eyes. This took place on a Tuesday, in the forenoon; and in the evening of the

same day he was so much worse that he was quite unable to open his eyes, they remaining fast closed. On the Saturday following medical advice was had recourse to, and caustic was applied to the parts by the gentleman who was consulted. The application of caustic was repeated as many as ten times. No improvement resulted from this mode of treatment; and the mother was told that the child would in all probability be blind for life. He did not complain of pain, but could not bear the light, even when the eyes were closed. Matters remained in this state for two or three weeks, when the mother came to Tiverton to see her sister, by whom she was advised to apply to Mr. Capern. Mr. C. commenced making the passes on Tuesday, September 18th, 1849, and on the following Saturday the child was able to open his eyes for the first time since the attack. It continued to improve. The eyes remained open, and though they still appeared weak and sensitive to light, and the lids were partly drawn down, and there was a slight inflammatory redness about the eyes, the sight of the left eye to all appearance was fully restored; but he had no power of vision with the right eye.

The professional gentlemen to whom he was shewn in Tiverton were of opinion that the sight of the right eye was totally destroyed in consequence of the injudicious application of caustic.

5. WILLIAM WOTTON, yeoman, Cadeleigh, aged 67 years, had a swelling, or what is termed a "rising," in the left eye for three weeks, that affected his sight. He applied to surgeons at the Eye Infirmary, Exeter,

who gave him medicine and ointment. Failing to obtain relief, he named it to Mr. Capern, who, at one sitting, completely restored his sight. This took place about two years since, and he has never since been inconvenienced by a return of the complaint.

September 30th, 1849.

6. Elizabeth Allen, wife of John Allen, of Bickleigh, states that she was nearly blind through weakness for four years. For twelve months she could not read or thread a needle without spectacles. The sight of the left eye was nearly lost. After a few applications to Mr. Capern she found herself able, on returning home, to read the smallest print, and even to thread a needle without spectacles. Her sight is now perfectly restored.

7. Eliza Quick, Townsend, Tiverton, aged 14 years, was subject from her sixth year to frequent and severe attacks of inflammation of the eyes, attended with great pain and injury to the sight. She seldom passed a month without an attack; and it often lasted six weeks. Sometimes she was constrained to spend more than a fortnight of that time in one position. Her eyes were kept completely covered, as she could not bear the least light. Many medical men were consulted both in Tiverton and Exeter, but without benefit. At the Eye Infirmary of the latter place her mother was informed that her daughter's case was quite hopeless at present. A change for the better, it was thought, might perhaps take place in her 15th year. At length

Mr. Capern was applied to; and after the very first mesmerisation there was a decided improvement: the pain was greatly alleviated, and by three or four applications she was completely cured. Nearly three years have elapsed since her cure, and there has been no return of the complaint. She is now apprenticed to a dressmaker.

Tiverton, October 4th, 1849.

8. SARAH PULSFORD, Andrew's Street, Tiverton, was attacked about two years since by a severe inflammation of the eye. She suffered intense pain, and could obtain but little or no sleep either by day or night. Her eye was much inflamed, having the appearance (to use her own expression) of a piece of 'raw liver.' She was confined to her house for fourteen weeks, and to a darkened room for eleven. She placed herself under the care of a surgeon in the town, but without benefit. She could not see at all with her left eye, and the gentleman attending her was of opinion that the sight on that side was permanently destroyed. Despairing of obtaining relief from ordinary remedies, and hearing much of Mr. Capern's cures, she was induced to request his attendance. She was in dreadful agony when he came; but, after he had operated upon her for about ten minutes, the pain was almost entirely removed and she was able to see a little. The second operation was attended by the complete disappearance of pain and by further improvement in her power of vision. She was afterwards mesmerised ten or twelve times more, and continued decidedly to improve. After the last

operation she was completely cured, and has not since had the slightest return of the pain.

October 17th, 1849.

9. JOHN HAWKINGS, aged 12 years, son of Susan Hawkings, Martin's Lane, Tiverton, caught a severe cold when on the line of march, at the age of 1 year, that settled in the eyelids, which became swollen and inflamed, discharging constantly a quantity of humour. After some time the eyes also became affected, and within three years, notwithstanding the best medical advice, the child became nearly blind—a thick dark film forming over each eye. In this state he continued until his twelfth year, gradually getting worse. At this time his heart became affected and he suffered much from palpitation, and was so weak that he would frequently fall without any apparent cause, remaining insensible for an hour. His mother, having experienced great relief from Mr. Capern's treatment, applied to that gentleman in behalf of her son; and he attended him daily for nearly ten months; at the end of which time the boy was perfectly cured. He derived benefit even at the commencement of the treatment. After being mesmerised daily for about four months, he was put almost daily into a sleep-waking state, and allowed to remain so until he waked of his own accord. He could latterly be entranced by his mother merely putting a bottle of mesmerised water into his hand. It ought to be mentioned that this boy was a patient of the Eye Infirmaries of both Bristol and Exeter.

10. Mrs. WARREN, wife of Mr. Warren of the Red Lion Inn, Tiverton, experienced severe affection of the eyes for several months, and for the three months previous to being operated upon she was in agonies of pain and was apprehensive she would lose the sight of both eyes. At the suggestion of several friends she applied to Mr. Capern, and after three sittings was completely cured. This took place nearly three years since, and there has been no return of the complaint since.

Red Lion Inn, Tiverton,
January 14th, 1851.

12. JOHN TEESDALE, a native of Yorkshire, but now a settler in Somerset, Niagara County, New York, had the misfortune, fourteen years ago, to have both eyes most severely injured (more particularly the left) by the bursting of a bottle of aqua fortis, a part of which entering his eyes caused the most excruciating pain and a high degree of inflammation. He was attended by three medical men at the same time, and continued under medical treatment for a period of eight years; during six of which they were in constant attendance upon him. He was cupped regularly three or four times a week for three months, and had seven blisters on him daily for a like period. He was also bled from the arm profusely, so as to induce fainting. On one occasion some pints of blood were taken from him, and used when cold as a poultice to the eyes. The left eye was in so deplorable a state that the doctors never gave him any hope of sight being restored to it, but confined their at-

tention to the right, being the better of the two. Among the remedies used, in addition to the above, during the last two years of the medical treatment, were the following,—lunar caustic, corrosive sublimate, blue and white vitriol. He had also snuff, burnt alum, loaf sugar, and powdered glass, blown into his eyes, with several other remedies. Sometimes the glass was mixed with a cerate and used as an ointment. He was under the treatment of no less than seventy-five medical men, having visited the following places in order to consult oculists of celebrity, viz., Flycreek, Cooperstown, Finstown, Utica, Geneva, Canandaigua, Schoharie, Buffalo, Albany Junction, Kingstown, New York, Toronto, Nidby, Upper Canada, Canton, Rome, Syracuse, and Somerset; but he derived no benefit whatever, remaining totally blind, and the right eye being quite destroyed by the remedies used, and the lid closed on an empty socket. He, therefore, for the last six years previous to his coming to England, gave up doctors and treated himself. In the autumn of 1849 he returned to England for the purpose of consulting some of the London oculists, but first went into Devonshire to visit some friends from whom he had been parted more than twenty years. Early in the month of November last, when on his way to London, he stopped at an inn (Red Lion) in Tiverton, and the landlady informed him that she herself had suffered from bad eyes, but had been cured by Mr. Capern, and urgently recommended him to visit that gentleman before he proceeded any further. After some enquiry he was induced to place himself under Mr. C.'s care, who mesmerised him two or three times a day for the first two months; and, extraordinary to relate, he derived benefit from the very first mesmeric operation, though only of about five minutes' duration. Mr. C. took him to Dr. Gervis, an oculist of Tiverton, who told them it was in vain to attempt anything with his eye, as it was beyond the power of mortal man to restore the sight, nearly the whole of the cornea being covered with a thick white film. Notwithstanding this damper upon his hopes, Mr. C. determined to persevere, and his success has surpassed their utmost expectations, as Teesdale can now read the signs over the shop doors, distinguish articles in the windows, and walk to any part of the town in perfect safety. The film is not removed, but the patient feels satisfied that it will be so eventually, and regrets that his means will not admit of his staying longer in this country. This patient is a man of Herculean strength and stature, and of strong nerve; yet has become so susceptible to the mesmeric influence that his mesmerist can place him, at any time, in a state of deep coma by merely holding one of his thumbs for less than ten seconds. This case being altogether so extraordinary and incredible, Mr. Capern deemed it prudent to have the above statement verified by the patient upon oath before Mr. Coles, a magistrate of the borough of Tiverton, as the patient could not hereafter be referred to, since he was about to return to America.

SECTION XI.

LOSS OF VOICE, THROAT & CHEST COMPLAINTS.

1. JEMIMA ACLAND, aged 73 years, had been poorly for a few days about two months ago, when she suddenly lost her voice, and could not speak above a whisper. At the end of six weeks she was advised by her daughter to send for Mr. Capern and be mesmerised, as the daughter herself had had her voice restored by that gentleman when lost in a similar manner. She did so; and, on his making a few mesmeric passes on her throat and chest, her voice was quite restored in five minutes. Her general health was also much improved.

2. ELIZABETH ZELLEY, aged 51 years, daughter of the above, caught a severe cold, and, in consequence, lost her voice, and had great difficulty in making herself heard. At the end of about eight weeks she was advised by her neighbours to apply to Mr. Capern. This she did the more readily in consequence of the wonderful cure performed by him on her own son; but she had no idea, until her neighbours mentioned it, that mesmerism could be useful in her case. Happening accidentally to meet Mr. Capern when on her way to his house, he desired her to accompany him into a neighbouring house,

and then, making a few passes on her throat and breast, completely restored her voice, much to the astonishment of all present.

3. HARRIETT, the wife of John T. Teesdale, in consequence of taking a severe cold about five months since, totally lost her voice; and this was followed by a swelling in the calf of the leg, that continued about three weeks. She was attended by a surgeon and a physician; the latter of whom advised her to go to bed, as it was necessary to have rest. They gave her medicine, and ordered a poultice to be applied to the swelling. The surgeon thought she would not be able to do anything for some time. This was on a Wednesday; but she, wishing to continue to work as long as possible, did not give up until the Saturday. A nurse was sent for to attend her. Mr. Capern was also sent for by her aunt, and in less than half a minute after his arrival she was in a state of mesmeric coma. Whilst in that state the passes were made with the palm of the hand over the chest and stomach, when an improvement of the voice was at once perceptible; and in less than ten minutes she could speak as well as ever. The passes were also made five or six times over the leg. The swelling subsided, the pain left her, and she resumed her work on the Wednesday following, and has never felt a return of the complaint from that time.

SECTION XII.

AFFECTIONS OF THE HEART.

1. ALICE DAVEY, Bampton, aged 50 years, mother of ten children, states that she has been suffering upwards of nineteen years from palpitation of the heart, accompanied with extreme weakness. She applied to different medical gentlemen, who assured her that they could in no way relieve her. She had also taken a variety of medicines recommended by different persons for the disease, but which did not at all benefit her. At length she was induced to apply to Mr. Thomas Capern, who made a few passes over the heart and side. The result was speedy relief. A cure was effected, and she is now as well as ever she was.

This statement was made three weeks after she was mesmerised, in the presence of A. Alderman, Esq., surgeon.

2. GEORGE SHOPLAND, residing at Cadbury, in the employ of Mr. Rew, surveyor of highways.—"I was taken ill in June, 1848, and was incapable of labour for three months; but although weak and unwell I continued to labour, except during the time named, until the spring of 1849, when I was compelled to wholly relinquish work. I had applied to a surgeon, who told me

it was a disease of the heart and asthma, that nothing would do me good, but advised my going to the Exeter Hospital. Instead of doing so, I applied to a medical gentleman of Exeter, who at first gave me relief; after which I became worse. I was then advised to apply to Mr. Capern, and the first time the passes were made over the stomach and heart I found great relief. On my seventh visit I felt confident of the result, and on the following day I was enabled to resume my labour of quarrying stone for Mr. Rew. Even without his touching me I experienced great sensations from Mr. C.'s hand being drawn over the affected part."

The surgeon who attended George Shopland appeared before the magistrates at Tiverton and made an affidavit that his complaints were disease of the heart and asthma, and that they would produce permanent disability.

3. William Zelley, son of the last mentioned person, now in his 10th year, came home from play about two years ago, complaining of a pain in the side and difficulty in breathing, accompanied with faintness. His father put his hand on the boy's heart and found it was palpitating fast and strongly. He continued getting worse for a week, when his mother sent for a doctor who attended him for some time, but without any beneficial result. At the end of a month a physician was consulted, who prescribed medicines, which he took for nearly three months: but he continued getting worse, and had become very pale and emaciated, and scarcely able to walk across the room. Indeed, so ill was he at this time that the doctors ordered him to be carried

when it became necessary to move him. The palpitation of the heart was frequently so great as to cause the bed in which he lay to vibrate, and its motion was visible to any one in the room. At this time his mother was advised by Mrs. Taylor and Mrs. Turner, two neighbours who had both been cured by Mr. Capern, to apply to him to mesmerise her boy. She did so, and he was mesmerised ten minutes daily for a month. He improved from the first visit of Mr. C., and at the end of the two months the complaint was entirely removed, and he walked a distance of four miles and a half without experiencing any bad effects. He remained so susceptible to mesmeric influence that a look from his mesmeriser would send him to sleep.

SECTION XIII.

AFFECTIONS OF THE STOMACH.

1. Henry Baker, of Hay-Park Farm, aged 40 years, about three years since became subject to severe pains in the pit of the stomach, and for the last twelve months they disabled him from labour. He applied to many medical men, had recourse to a variety of remedies, and was for some time at the Exeter Hospital, and also under the treatment of an eminent physician of that city; but all without the least relief. He was brought very low by the remedies applied, and was reduced to so weak a state that he was scarcely able to go about at all, even in the house. His debility and emaciation were so great that he was considered by his family, as well as himself, to be in a decline. In this condition he was advised to apply to Mr. Capern. He found immediate relief from the contact passes of the palm of the hand down the front of the body. After three operations of ten minutes each he was free from all pain. This took place about two years since. Two months after the last operation had been performed Mr. Capern met him in the street, and finding, upon enquiry, that he was suffering from a slight attack of his old complaint, in consequence, as he believes, of having over-reached himself whilst engaged in his employment, which is la-

borious and requires at times a great exertion of muscular force, offered to operate upon him, and with a few passes entirely removed the pain. Since then it has never returned, and he is now quite well and strong, attends regularly to his employment, and is capable of performing a good day's work without fatigue or inconvenience. His expenses for medicine, &c., previously to applying to Mr. Capern, were about £30, and from that time it has not been five shillings.

December, 1849.

2. Statement of Mr. JOHN OXENHAM, yeoman, Bampton.

"I had been ill above seven years with severe pains in the head and stomach; and it was the general opinion of various professional gentlemen whom I consulted at Bampton, Wiveliscombe, Tiverton, and Taunton, that they were occasioned by a weakness of the digestive organs. The only point on which they disagreed was, as to the probability of a permanent cure. One of them—an eminent physician—asserted that nothing would ever benefit me; whilst others were of a contrary opinion. By all of them, however, the strictest attention to diet was declared to be indispensably necessary; and they invariably advised my discontinuing the use of vegetables, which direction I carefully complied with, as experience shewed me the advantage of it. By a rigid adherence to those rules I suffered considerably less pain and inconvenience after eating; yet, in spite of the quantity of medicine which I took, there was no improvement in my health. At length, believing my case to be hopeless,

I abstained entirely from taking medicine. Whilst in this state I was induced, by the many reports I had heard of the cures effected by Mr. Capern, to apply to him. After the first passes were made over the head and stomach I felt much better. I have since been operated upon three times, at intervals of some weeks: and now, thanks to Mr. C. for his exertions, consider myself cured. The time occupied in making the respective passes was from ten minutes to a quarter of an hour. I first applied to Mr. Capern about five months since.

"October 21st, 1849."

SECTION XIV.

EMACIATION AND DEBILITY IN CHILDREN.

1. JOHN GIBBINGS, aged nearly 5 years, when first seen by Mr. Capern, was very weak and emaciated. His shoulder blades were almost protruding through the skin; and, being unable to stand alone, he passed the whole of the day either in his cradle or propped up in a chair. Before removing to Tiverton his parents had resided at Plymouth, and the child had been attended by three of the most eminent physicians of that place since he was twelve months old, but without benefit. He was also under the care of different surgeons of Tiverton. Mr. Capern, commiserating the poor child's case on seeing the deplorable condition to which he was reduced, resolved to try the effects of mesmerism. And the following is the satisfactory result. A slight improvement in the child's health was observable after the third or fourth operation. At the end of six weeks he was able to walk. Mr. C. continued his mesmeric operations daily for two months longer, and then saw him less frequently. At the end of seven months his health was quite restored, and he is now quite a fine spirited little fellow. At one time the child was so ill that the nurse called his mother to close his eyes, as she considered him dying.

2. Richard Thorne, son of John Thorne, tinman, St. Andrew's Street, aged 3½ years, had been very weak and sickly from his birth, his body being much swollen, particularly on the left side. His appetite was good. His mother consulted a surgeon and physician, but without any beneficial result. They gave her no hope of improvement, and considered him dropsical. Just before completing his second year he became weaker than ever, was unable to stand, and with difficulty sat in a chair supported by pillows, and only felt ease by lying on his back. This was his state when Mr. Capern first operated upon him. After the first mesmerisation he began to improve, and was able to stand alone at the end of a week. He was attended by Mr. C. for about a month, being operated upon two or three times a week; and at the expiration of six weeks could walk alone, and is now a strong healthy child—a year and a half having expired since he was first visited by Mr. Capern.

FINIS.

Walton & Mitchell, Printers, 24, Wardour Street, London.

Spotted something that isn't quite right?

Let us know and we'll fix it for future reprints. And as a thank you for your diligence, we'll send you a free Sothis book of your choice.

publisher@sothis.press

This page intentionally left blank

Except of course for that line above. And this one.
And whilst we have your attention, perhaps you'd
like to follow us on Instagram @sothis.press. Go on.

Made in the USA
Monee, IL
08 November 2026

67983442R00090